Essays From The Couch

By

William S. Horowitz M.D.

Copyright © 2011 William S. Horowitz M.D.
All rights reserved.

ISBN: 1456468944
ISBN-13: 9781456468941

Library of Congress Control Number: 2010919647

TABLE OF CONTENTS

FOREWARD	VII
DEDICATION	IX
ACKNOWLEDGEMENTS	XI
PREFACE I	XIII

PART I

ACTING AND ACTING OUT: A FRAGMENT	1
A.D.D.: AN UNORTHODOX APPROACH	3
INTRODUCTION	5
INCIDENCE AND ASSOCIATED CONDITIONS	7
HISTORY AND SYMPTOMATOLOGY	9
PHYSICAL MARKERS	13
ETIOLOGY	15
THERAPY	17
RESISTANCE TO THERAPY	21
DIFFERENTIAL DIAGNOSIS	25
PROGNOSIS	27
PROFESSIONAL ADDENDUM PSYCHODYNAMICS OF ADD	31
A PSYCHOANALYST LOOKS AT ALCOHOLICS ANONYMOUS (ADDENDUM IV)	37
"AS-IF" PERSONALITY: A CLINICAL CAUTION	41
"THE BOOTSTRAPPERS": A CONTEMPORARY CHARACTEROLOGY	45
THUMBNAIL SKETCH OF THE BORDERLINE PATIENT	83
THE CENTRAL NERVOUS SYSTEM AND BEHAVIOR,	89
DISCUSSION OF THE TREATMENT OF NARCISSISTIC DISORDERS BY DR. BURNESS MOORE	91
DISCUSSION OF NORMAL AND PATHOLOGICAL NARCISSISM BY DR. OTTO KERNBERG	99

DISCUSSION OF DEFENSIVE AVOIDANCE OF PRIMARY IDENTITY BY DR. MAURICE WALSH	103
DISCUSSION OF PSYCHOANALYSTS & PSYCHOANALYTIC EDUCATION BY DR. ROBERT DORN	107
EMBATTLED PSYCHIATRY	111
HELPFUL HINTS FROM HOROWITZ	115
HOMOSEXUALITY	119
WHAT WE DON'T SPEAK ABOUT: HUMAN AGGRESSION	121
NARCISSISM	
SUPERIOR BEING	133
TOWARD A UNIFYING CONCEPTION OF NARCISSISM	137
"PITFALLS OF THERAPY"	165
SEXUAL ADDICTION	181
WORK-DOES THE PATIENT HAVE TO WORK ?	185
POSTSCRIPT	189

PART II

AN ESSAY ON JEWISH ATAVISM AND THEOCRACY	191
JEWS IV	231
LETTER TO DR. BREINER	235
LETTER TO DR. STEIN	237
THE SIGNIFICANCE OF 4 YEARS	241
SPECULATIONS	245
WASP-A PROTESTANT DISEASE, AMERICAN GOTHIC, OR THE STATE OF WASPISHNESS.	259

PART III

BOOBUS AMERICANUS II	281
CITIZENSHIP-GULLIVER IN IRAQ	283
COMPETITION II	285
DEMOGRAPHICS	289

DEPENDENCY	291
DIAMOND IN THE ROUGH	295
DUTY	297
THE EQUIVALENCE GAME	299
THE "EXPERIMENT" HAS FAILED	301
THE GESTURE	303
GREED – 8/28/08	305
GREED II – 8/30/08	309
GROW UP, ALREADY	311
HELMETS	313
HOLIDAZE	317
INTEGRATION	319
INTIMACY	323
IT'S NOT FAIR !	325
JUDGMENT	327
TO THE LETTERS TO THE EDITOR	329
MY PASSAGE	331
ON ACHIEVING PERSONHOOD	333
PLAY	335
POLY SCI 101	337
POME	339
POWER	341
REFLECTIONS	345
RIGHTEOUSNESS	349
THE SCOURGE OF THE TWENTIETH CENTURY	351
SHAME ON YOU	355
SURVIVOR GUILT	357
THE POLITICS OF SEX	359
TO BE OR NOT TO BE	361
TO BELONG	365
WOMEN	367

FOREWARD

William S. Horowitz, M.D.
November 1, 2010

I am proud, dear reader, to present for your consideration some of the ideas gleaned from my psychoanalytic practice of some 55 years. I am 86 now, wanting to leave something of value to my family, patients, friends and colleagues, to all of whom I owe a debt of gratitude for their support and teachings.

A brief professional biography might be in order. I attended the Shorewood school system, then on to the University of Wisconsin and Dartmouth College as an undergraduate; University of Chicago School of Medicine '44 to '49, in part in Naval uniform; Barnes Hospital St. Louis and University of Cincinnati for Psychiatric residency, in part in Air Force uniform; '54 enrolled in Los Angeles Psychoanalytic Institute, graduated circa '59; had one training analysis, then a later therapeutic one with another analyst, the known names of whom I will not drop, but to whom I am deeply indebted; appointed Training and Supervising Analyst and headed several committees in the Society in due course. I practiced mostly therapeutic analysis in Beverly Hills (chiefly Hollywood professionals) and Palos Verdes (chiefly physicians); practiced psychiatry in the military and Palm Springs.

These essays are grouped as clinical, sociological, and free ranging thoughts on diverse subjects. They owe their inspiration to the rich stimulation and learning I received from my patients and their treatments, hence titled, "Essays from the Couch". I hope the clinical situation rewarded them as much as me.

DEDICATION

To my mother for her nurturance and my education, to my father and his father before him for breaking the chains of conformity, to my sister for her protection and acculturation of her kid brother, to my wife for her sustaining me and my productivity in my senescence, to all our children and their children, and in memory of those beloveds who left our family before their time.

ACKNOWLEDGEMENTS

This work would not have been possible without the loving and dedicated efforts of my friend, Philip Bronner, MD, his invaluable assistant Kelly Talbot and my wife, Gloria. The ideas would not have been possible without the productive work of innumerable patients, honoring the invention of Sigmund Freud.

PREFACE I

This is a collection of (mostly oral) essays which were prepared over the course of my psychoanalytic career, and, as I can see now, on one topic. The early papers are included more for their historical than expository value, reflecting as they do my own as well as contemporary evolving conceptualizations in the field about the subject matter.

The chief evolution in my orientation has been a developing dissatisfaction with the concept of "normal" narcissism, clarification of the distinction between shame and guilt (ego-ideal vs. super-ego tension), shifting of the focus in the phenomenon of acting-out from an historical, transference perspective to one of a reaction to being dealt with by a narcissistic partner, and the replacement of the concept of symbiosis with parasitism. From the beginning, I have conceived of narcissism as both a stage of normal childhood psychic development interposed between the preceding fusion stage and succeeding separate-object relationship stage, and in the adult, as a mode of relating constituting a dynamic defense against separate-object relationships. Accompanying this perspective has been a shift in focus from the traditional libidinal point of view to one of the predominance of aggressive instinctual phenomena.

These developmental and defensive states antedate the capacity for classical transference, and therefore modify the applicability of classical psychoanalytic technique to their understanding and treatment. The resulting confusion and misapprehensions about the fate of narcissistic strivings in our theory, as well as its strong intrinsic resistance to therapeutic modification, have led to a tolerance of unanalyzed residua in our patient population and particularly our psychoanalytic trainees, with a consequent unfortunate persistence of unilateral rather than reciprocal transactions in our technique and our professional institutions, which make the understanding and treatment of this pathology all the more problematic.

Preface I

Actual derivatives of childhood narcissism are manifold, their qualification qua derivatives depending on the degree of sublimation of the original energy (de-instinctualization, aim and object change, fusion, and binding), which is always subject to both incomplete transformation and regressive de-differentiation (as in nightly regression into sleep and in the state of illness). In addition, sublimated self-libido can be admixed in varying degrees with object-libido, making its tracing even more disguised. This very profusion of repositories for infantile narcissism, this ubiquity, is one of the factors which lends support to the perception of its "normalcy" in adulthood, which in turn is one of the many masks narcissism can wear.

These derivatives may include but are not limited to investments in: adult love-objects, our women and children, as well as separate objects in general; our heroes, gods, religions, nations, polities, organizations, and institutions; our character defenses (armor of Reich) and its sense of identity; our self (ego-feeling of Federn), its esteem and its wishes (dreams); our ego-ideal and its aspirations (fantasies); our home, clothes, photos, memories and memorabilia, personal possessions; our tastes, values, habits, personal ideas and philosophy, speech and writing; our skills, talents, and profession; our artistic creations, scientific discovery and invention; our body and its parts, grooming of and care for its health; our life in both its experiential, contextual and biographic, reflexive mode; fantasies of after-life survival; and, our actual after-life legacy to our survivors.

I acknowledge my indebtedness to all who have patiently taught me, from my parents and extended family, through all my professional teachers from early school years on through the psychoanalytic institute, my personal analysts, the professor and the multiplicity of psychoanalytic authors who followed him, and all my patients, the treatment situation with them having been a constant stimulus to new ideas. I could not have done without the support I have received from my wife and son, and those many others who have critiqued my work and encouraged me to proceed. Nor could I have managed this piece-by-piece assemblage without my computer at the ready directly from the consultation room. And lastly, I am grateful to my publisher for this forum.

ACTING AND ACTING OUT: A FRAGMENT

"All the world's a stage, and all the people in it merely players." Mature social behavior involves a hierarchical series of successful identifications (each of which starts, however, with a role assigned and accepted), combining to form an identity, which then permits the adoption of a series of discrete roles in different contexts in which one "acts" appropriate to the role. In this sense, normal behavior involves acting, and what we term "acting-out" involves not acting, not playing the social game. It is a primitive attempt to contact an object and gain discharge, utilizing partially unbound and defused energies for unsublimated aims.

Chronic actor-outers were, and often still are, the objects of acting-out on the part of their parents. Typically, the parent, often the mother, a narcissistic infantile guilt-ridden person herself, relates to the child as herself, filling the child with projected impulses and guilts, and also as a transference figure from her own past, sibling, and/or parent. In either case, the child well appreciates his not being treated as himself, and acutely senses the absence of contact. (This, I believe, is the basis of the clinical phenomenon of acting-out on the part of the patient when the analyst misses an interpretation, loses contact with his patient, often on the basis of his transferences or projections. The patient then immediately regresses and attempts to regain contact, not the least of which is by curbing from the analyst. This is entirely analogous to a "misunderstood" child.)

In addition to the conventional acting-out described above, these patients, out of compliance to their mother's needs and out of regression away from violent Oedipal conflicts, act the role of a helpless infant, while relating to mother and her surrogates, while to a large extent normal ego development continues and flourishes in secret, often in relation to healthier objects (usually selected teachers).

AN UNORTHODOX APPROACH TO ADULT ATTENTION DEFICIT DISORDER (A.D.D.)

A 1992-1996 PERSONAL TOUR OF DISCOVERY

PRESENTED AT THE A.P.A CONGRESS OF MAY 1996 AT WASHINGTON D.C.

William S. Horowitz, M.D.

INTRODUCTION

I first became aware of this disorder in adults after serving in child and adolescent hospitals in several states, then encountering for myself the identical picture in adult hospital and out-patient settings in yet other states. This discovery took place during my locum tenens travels around the country during the past 4 years, as with Rip Van Winkle after my retirement from 40 years of an entirely different type of psychiatric practice.

This interest was compelled by the striking prevalence of this disorder in my clinical work. It did not spring from readings in the American psychiatric literature or teachings from academia, but rather the necessity to treat live patients at the bedside. Hence my approach is not the traditional one, but it has been forged in the rigorous necessities of clinical practice.

I attended a lecture three years ago by a neurologist specializing in this disorder which confirmed my observations and verified that the clinical syndrome in adults then had increasing acceptance as existing. Readings in the foreign literature, much more open to new ideas, also served to confirm my experiences. I will speak to you about my own clinical findings now with over 1000 cases, rather than attempting to review the current literature which is beginning to emerge and overflow.

INCIDENCE AND ASSOCIATED CONDITIONS

The disorder is more prevalent than thought, not at all rare. In most settings, I have seen several cases a week, sometimes a day, usually undiagnosed or misdiagnosed as manic-depression ("Bipolarity"), major depression ("Unipolarity"), or mood instability secondary to drug abuse (which is usually vice versa); on rare occasions, the diagnosis of mental retardation has been given to an illiterate but intelligent patient, or psychosis to an inarticulate but intelligent patient.

On the other hand, beware of a fad diagnosis of labeling everyone with this. It is a well-defined disorder, with limits, which you will learn as you become more familiar with it. In the adult it is typically found in the context of anxiety, depression and substance abuse, past or present, and can occur in conjunction with P(ost) T(raumatic) S(tress) D(isorder), Panic Disorder, Obsessive-Compulsive Disorder, Intermittent Explosive Disorder, Conduct Disorder, Personality Disorder, Borderline Disorder, Learning Disorder, and Dyslexia, and has a special association (70%) with Giles de la Tourette's Syndrome. The historic name for the disorder was M(inimal) B(rain) D(ysfunction). The future name might well be Neurotransmitter Deficiency Disorder, or possibly Cerebral Immaturity.

An incidental paradoxical finding is that not a few of the undiagnosed and untreated patients come from families where the parents are educators, psychologists, or physicians. These are people whom one would assume would be aware of this disorder; possibly the explanation lies in the occurrence of the disorder in the parent also which may blind him to its abnormality.

The relationship of the childhood to the adult form of the disorder is variable. Most children with ADD progress directly into the adult form; some have their symptoms attenuate or disappear in adulthood; and very rarely adult forms seem to spring de novo without an antecedent history.

There also may be gender differences: some boys tend to be hyperactive and read, write, and speak poorly; some girls tend to be day-dreamers and love to read phantasy material, but calculate and read "hard" material poorly.

HISTORY AND SYMPTOMATOLOGY

The condition is characterized by disordered perceptions, thinking, memory, emotions, and conduct. Behaviorally, the patients are typified by impatience, inattentiveness, impulsivity, and irritability. They often have a variable educational history (sometimes poor, sometimes compensatory outstanding, sometimes both: high school drop-out followed by straight A's in later college) and unstable employment and marital record in the presence often of high intelligence and creativity, and a tendency in adolescence and young adulthood toward substance abuse, delinquency, and an unusual incidence of auto accidents.

You will learn to recognize as pathognomonic flags: (1) such expressions from the patients as, "I'm not normal; I'm different; I'm not stupid". Other clues in the history-taking suggesting more detailed inquiry are: (2) childhood learning disability with special education or reading classes; (3) childhood hyperactivity (restlessness, class disruption and fighting), with or without diagnosis and treatment, in the patient or his close relatives; (4) history of self-medication often starting in adolescence, with stimulants (caffeine, amphetamines, cocaine), sedatives (marijuana, alcohol, rarely heroin), or prescribed anxiolytics (benzodiazopenes) or antidepressants (SSRIs); (5) history of a paradoxical reaction to medication (stimulation from sedatives; sedation from stimulants); (6) history of childhood physical abuse, which may stem from an overwhelmed parent mal-coping with an uncontrolled child rather than a primarily uncontrolled parent (or, they both may be); (7) unusually poor spelling in the presence of a college degree; (8) stuttering or pseudo-blocking in the giving of the history; (9) scattering of thoughts and disorganization of the narrated history, resembling a thought disorder; (10) and inarticulate speech resembling pseudo-stupidity in a patient with otherwise good intelligence (e.g. vocabulary).

The perceptual/cognitive disorder must be inquired into in detail, for it may be unrecognized by them. If asked specifically, they will confirm that they must read or listen to material several times to "get it", having trouble taking it in, comprehending it, retaining and recalling it. Some can take in by ear what they cannot by eye, or vice versa. Many describe the words as "running together, floating away," or "having no meaning". They cannot sit through a protracted lecture, film, book, newspaper article, or conversation without getting up to "take a break". Very typically they will interrupt others' talking, and are often accused of not listening. They find it difficult to articulate a coherent line of thought. (One test developed for diagnosis is reading the patient a simple one-paragraph story; they cannot reproduce it.)

They are afraid they cannot learn new ideas, whether conveyed by written or oral words or diagrams, to learn to operate new machinery, follow new procedures, or find their way by instruction. The former gives rise to failure to advance on the job for years, the latter to getting lost and a travel phobia or pseudo-agoraphobia. Many describe their inability to focus in general because of either a "fog" or a profusion of distracting thoughts (which often prevent sleep), although paradoxically may be able to overcompensate and concentrate on a subject of high interest to them. The patients typically will have a number of unfinished projects, jobs, or relationships, not to mention unstarted ones, as they complain they "can never do anything right" or "finish anything", reflecting also their demoralized self-esteem.

They are subject to extreme emotional lability, which they can describe by gesture as following a jagged, irregular pattern rather than a smooth alternation of mood, although they may use the popular and inaccurate term "mood-swings" to describe it. The content of the mood ranges from happy to sad, calm to angry and irritable, sober to frivolous, typically "shifting on a dime". The lability is in part not spontaneous but in reaction to extreme frustration with their ineffective cognition and action (and the inability of anyone to diagnose and treat them properly), in part a product of accumulated undischarged tension. This chronic tension frequently gives rise to somatic symptoms in the adult, such as muscular back, neck, head, and joint pain. In youngsters, on the other hand, the tension is typically discharged through vigorous physical exercise in sports.

The patients are also highly subject to boredom, another cause of shifting interests, and seek excitement through counterphobic risk-taking, another self-treatment through psychic rather than drug stimulation. The peak in their frustration is usually manifested by either a build-up of tension to the point of explosive discharge, in phantasy or action, or fitful (short-lived) episodes of extreme despondency, often accompanied by a serious suicide attempt.

PHYSICAL MARKERS

There may be present "soft" neurological signs such as strabismus, stuttering, tics, minor tremors or choreo-athetoid movements, myoclonic jerks, clumsiness, or generalized restlessness often evident during the examination, sometimes only during or surrounding sleep. The strabismus, often first manifested in childhood and "corrected", may give rise to the symptom of inability to focus (an interesting physical correlate to the psychic one) with a "lazy eye", suppression of the image in that eye, and loss of depth perception. This, plus inattentiveness, impatience, impulsivity, and failure to learn constitute a dangerous mixture on the road resulting in frequent automobile collisions.

Characteristically, during the interview a part of the adult patient's body (a foot, e.g.) will have its motor running, will "idle" (origin of the term "shake a leg?"), which they recognize as a life-long habit, and which you can recognize as THE pathognomonic sign. The typical motion is one foot with its toes on the floor, its heel lifted, pumping or bouncing the heel up and down at a rapid tempo. You can make this diagnosis long-distance even before starting the examination. This sign is the external manifestation of the subjective tension which some describe as a "live wire" (origin of the term "wired"?). In children the whole body is restless and cannot sit still through the interview, either rocking or getting up out of the chair to wander the examination room.

ETIOLOGY

There were over 1,200 citations in the international literature in the 6 years up through 1995, France and New Zealand leading the foreign sources, most of them concerning the childhood version. Highlights of over 300 of these papers follow:

Research has identified a state of cortical hypoarousal in these patients with a compensatory over-activation, and an asymmetry in size of the bilateral heads of the caudate nuclei (L<R) opposite to that found normally (L>R). They also have been demonstrated to have a modification in their hypothalamic-pituitary-adrenal axis (abnormal diurnal rhythm, non-suppression to DST), and to be resistant to thyroid hormone. Foods and additives have been demonstrated to be causal in some cases. There is a definite genetic component to the disorder (the gene recently having been identified), and most often one of the parents can retrospectively be identified as having had it, as well as one of the patient's siblings or children. (One patient may turn into 2 or 3.)

With the apparent burgeoning of the world-wide incidence of this disorder in recent years, one's curiosity is naturally aroused as to possible 20th century etiologic agents. The literature remains silent on this subject, except for excluding certain factors, which area would seem to be ripe for exploration.

In my personal experience, certain populations of ADD patients have a majority with an asthmatic/allergic diathesis; this is especially intriguing when one realizes that tricyclics, which most of these patients respond to, were originally synthesized as anti-histamine agents. And, in fact, the asthma or ticking cough itself is often alleviated as well in therapy.

THERAPY

Treatment historically has been by stimulants such as Ritalin, Cylert, and amphetamines. Ritalin has many problems, including being a controlled substance (recently discovered to having been sold and abused in the schoolyard), not inexpensive, suppressing appetite and retarding growth in youngsters, being very short-acting thus leading to rapid cycling, and having earned a bad reputation from unsatisfactory results which either deters many families from starting treatment or has them quit shortly. Never-the-less and amazingly, it alone seems to have been anointed as the drug of choice in this country.

Newer agents include tricyclic and serotonergic antidepressants, which are preferred in many other countries. My favorite of these by far is imipramine HCl which I call the "magic" medicine, which is well tolerated after the third or fourth day, very effective at low doses not requiring blood levels or EKGs, single bed-time dosage, without serious lasting side-effects, inexpensive, non-addictive, and controlling of the perceptual, cognitive, emotional, and behavioral aspects of the disorder and co-existing disorders all at the same time...thus rendering excellent compliance. Compliance is not exactly the word, for the medication is so relieving that the patients would not want to give it up (children typically will request their medicine before bed).

I usually prescribe 25 mgm. size pills to allow us to titrate to the optimum level, which finally is up to the patient to determine for himself. The usual final dose will fall between 75 and 125 mgms. at supper or bedtime in adults. Children and adolescents are more tolerant of higher doses of the drug (rarely experiencing side-effects) than middle-aged and older patients who may experience cerebral anti-cholinergic effects. One can start with 75, or with a loading dose of 100 (125 for adolescents or heavy adults) which will raise the blood level faster and minimize the initial side effects, then titrate up or down as needed. Some will benefit with an additional 25 in the morning if the effects wear off by late afternoon or evening. Unusually sensitive patients (those with low thresholds for medication in general) may do better on a gradual titration upwards from a low starting dose. Very small children (age 4+, weight 50#) do well on 25-50 mgms; seniors (ages 60-85) may benefit from 10-25 mgms.

Beneficial effects will usually be noted within days, but a minimum trial of 2 weeks is recommended for evaluation, and benefits continue to increase for months. Tolerance does not seem to develop; oppositely, sometimes the dose can be decreased over time (to 50 mgms.). Some patients discover that they can get along completely without it after some months, almost as though something has been "reset" in their brain chemistry.

Side effects appearing over the first 24-72 hours may include light-headedness upon arising, dry mouth, a feeling of "spaciness" or "walking on water", bladder or rectal hesitancy, sweating or heat-intolerance, or any idiosyncratic sensation. The patient should be reassured that continuing the medication will see these side-effects diminish significantly and the beneficial effects appear with the rise in blood level, often abruptly over one day. Dropping the dose at this early point only perpetuates the side-effects and aborts the beneficial ones, resulting in a frightened and unhappy patient who will quit. After the patient has stabilized in a week or two is the time to adjust the dosage down if there is 1) daytime sedation, or 2) forgetfulness, or 3) nighttime cessation of dreaming, or up if there is insufficient control: the leg-pumping or body-shaking tremor should disappear completely.

Imipramine's superior effectiveness to the amphetamines is probably due to the modification of three neurotransmitters rather than just one: the norepinephrine, dopamine, and serotonin systems. The patients will typically report that they sleep soundly, awaken energetic but calm, their mental "fog" has disappeared and they can think and read clearly, and they are emotionally stable, organized, and productive. You will notice their tremor has disappeared. Their families will tell them they are "a new person", or the "lovable old person" they have seen at times. Students and their teachers will note an immediate ability to complete their assignments, often after the first dose! After a week of medication many will report, "I'm normal for the first time in my life!".

Patients who are not true ADD will find the medication too stimulating and interfering with sleep and will stop it. However, this may be either a side-effect of low blood level, or the effect of inconsistent potency rather than a failure to respond; sometimes a few more days will see the desired outcome. There are now five generic manufacturers whose products are not standardized, by definition, and the clinical effects of each will vary from batch to batch and pharmacy to pharmacy, which you and your patient need to be aware of in regulating dosages. Brand-name Tofranil is not as consistently effective in all patients as the generic preparation for some reason; beware of the pharmacist "substituting upwards" for convenience, unbeknownst to you, and the patient suddenly not tolerating it. Second choice in treatment are any of the other tricyclics, which are less potent but also less side-effect producing; the two, imi- and desi-/other, can be mixed to alleviate persistent side-effects. Small doses of valproate can be added to control severe conduct disorder; miniscule amounts of Haldol will reduce some patients'(see below) hypersensitivity.

I am aware that a body of helpful non-medical measures, plus support groups, have developed over the years for assisting children with this disability. In adults, education and support can play a vital role in overcoming:

RESISTANCE TO THERAPY

This whole initiation of treatment process is relatively simple and straightforward in the youthful uncontaminated patient who has not yet accumulated significant secondary gain. Typically he will be delighted to find relief and the additional bonus that he is not mentally ill and will confirm it with, "I knew it!".

As might be expected, however, when a patient has carried a diagnosis of serious mental illness for years or decades, apparently confirmed by a succession of doctors and treated with industrial strength medication regimens, the introduction of the idea by a new doctor that he may not be a manic-depressive and may require only a simple treatment for relief can be met with disbelief, mistrust, anxiety, and confounding symptoms, particularly during the attempt to withdraw him from those medications. This is especially the case when he has been warned, "Never stop your Lithium!", has become addicted to benzodiazopines, or has become invalided and compensated for it.

This is a secondary level of resistance added on top of the primary: as could be expected from a symptom complex of inability to pay attention but the drawing of it from others, those with a co-existing personality disorder will often have narcissistic features, those with a conduct disorder a stubborn defiance of external control: the central psychodynamic feature of all seems to be a resistance to taking in. These psychological features, elaborated elsewhere, naturally do not disappear with treatment of the ADD, but may be profoundly altered by it.

This felt loss of control can be a powerful source of resistance by the patient becoming anxious about the newly-experienced absence of tension and withdrawing from treatment. This is typical of Borderline patients who need to maintain control, and may be found among a sub-set of middle-aged females who complain of idiosyncratic side-effects (probably representing dis-integration rather than a direct drug effect) which make this and all medications intolerable except for their favored benzodiazepines and street drugs. This is the sole group of patients in which the treatment may be contraindicated.

The implication of this work, of course, is that adult ADD by itself is a neurological disorder (perhaps somewhat analogous to a seizure disorder) and not a mental illness, unfortunately so far too often unrecognized by the psychiatrist who is the professional most often exposed to these cases, and by the mental health clinic and its staff which is the agency most often involved in funding treatment.

These professionals have their own resistance to treatment. There are psychological components to this disorder which can easily becloud its fundamental nature, and there is the inertia to new ideas which characterize humans and the bureaucracies they create, to name two sources, often manifested in a resistive group-think. In addition, it is entirely possible that there may be a philosophical motive for this non-recognition by the ancillary staff, who define their success in public agencies under the social work model of delivering services to the greatest number of clients and expending the largest number of dollars. Thus they may fear that the maintenance of a roster of "seriously mentally ill" clients is in jeopardy, that supply which is the source of its capitated (by the head-count) income not to mention its sense of usefulness and even its jobs. By contrast, and sometimes in explicit struggle, the physician who operates under the medical model is continually striving to restore his patient to autonomy, to eliminate the need for his own services.

This impetus to overtreatment, compensation, regression and chronicity is but an extension of the general dependency culture which has been created and perpetuated for decades for political, definitely not therapeutic, purposes. The practitioner who attempts to heal these patients and get them off the sick list is bucking both a formidable political and psychological opposition indeed, he should be warned, which may well target him as well as his cases. The support of the patient, family, professional staff, and administration of the agency are absolutely essential to successful treatment, which means educating them, and without it, the whole program will surely be sabotaged. But the rewards are considerable, also, especially from the grateful patients.[1]

The first appearance of side-effects the first or second day of treatment can mobilize this resistance for both patient and professional and provide the rationale for stopping it. When this hurdle is confronted, by explicit anticipation of these side effects, telephone monitoring and reassurance, however, this impediment can be overcome if the motivation to do so is present.

---

1 I have learned recently that certain school boards by policy deliberately avoid the recognition and referral of pupils with ADD for diagnosis and treatment so as to circumvent the contingent responsibility of providing special services to them. For similar reasons, certain county clinics will recognize and treat childhood ADD, but not adult, mistakenly fearing the expense of it. One national HMO will not compensate for an evaluation for ADD, but will for follow-up visits after the diagnosis is made. These bald financial motives well may be the major factor in the institutional resistance I have found so prevalent. A world-class substance abuse center eschews the diagnosis and treatment of ADD because of its religio-philosophical refusal to include any medication in its treatment program.

DIFFERENTIAL DIAGNOSIS

Those mis-diagnosed as manic depressive disorder ("Bipolarity") typically will have been treated vigorously with a variety of potent anti-manic and anti-psychotic preparations, those as depressive disorder ("Unipolarity") with potent anti-depressant preparations...all rendering small benefit and leading to many diagnosis and medication changes, a befogged and displeased patient, and a beclouded history. Usually you can establish a life-long thread of symptoms in the true ADD reaching back into early childhood, or at very least sometimes only in the patient's children or siblings.

M/D does not first appear at age 3 or 5; hyperness typically does. M/D does not make its first appearance in middle age. In ADD, there is no cyclicality, no true mania (2-3 days of round-the-clock activity), no protracted (weeks or months) depression, no strong family history of manic-depressive disorder, nor near-perfect control and patient satisfaction with lithium. In addition, the frequency of these disorders is quite different: ADD is very common, true M/D is not so common, certainly not as common as is diagnosed in the usual clinic setting where the recent popularization of the concept of "Bipolarity" and the practice of diagnosis-inflation may unfortunately combine to justify treatment. The question of whether these two conditions can coexist has been raised in only three cases in my series so far, therefore remains theoretical.

Those who doubt the prevalence of adult ADD have only to account for the fate of all the childhood cases which are flooding every clinic which I have witnessed in a veritable epidemic! Additionally, what could use further explanation are the puzzling frequencies of the diagnosis of "Bipolarity" and the prescribing of Lithium and Ritalin.

Single or recurrent major depressive disorders typically are not over in a few days, nor resolve spontaneously, but do respond favorably with either first or second generation anti-depressants. The ADD patient will report partial and temporary benefit only from that typical regimen.

Here is the diagnostic triad for adult ADD to take home with you: 1) a childhood history of reading disability, still present, 2) an adolescent preference for 'speed', and 3) an adult leg-shaking. When these three features are present, you can make the diagnosis with 99% confidence. This triad could be remembered as Read, Speed, and Feed(t). There are cases which you may learn to suspect as your experience grows where only one or two of this triad are present, or only a few of the manifold symptoms of the typical case, formes frustes if you will, which may warrant a diagnostic and therapeutic trial of imipramine. I have found such cases among the most seriously disturbed patients diagnosed as mentally defective or chronically psychotic; the fear and resistance to treatment by the clinic and family are proportionately highest in these rare instances.

Cases diagnosed as pure Learning Disorder, Dyslexia, Tourette's, Intermittent Explosive or Obessional Disorder merit a thorough work-up for ADD and probably a diagnostic trial of medication. From the clinical material presenting to me, I am beginning to doubt that they exist as isolated entities.

PROGNOSIS

It is most gratifying to see this truly curative result in the appropriate patient, a rarity in our psychiatric and medical practice, which, once witnessed, will convince you, the patient, and the staff of the validity of this syndrome as a discrete entity. This medication test thus serves as a validation of your clinical diagnosis, as does the patient discovering himself in this paper with the comment, "How did you know my secrets?". (I routinely hand out a version of this to patients considering undergoing treatment.)

I am not aware of long-term studies, since the recognition of this disorder in adults is recent. However, if bleeding or infections ensue, a WBC should be taken; arrhythmia, an EKG; signs of toxicity, a blood level. A low blood level is not significant, for this medication does not require the usual antidepressant therapeutic level for effectiveness in this condition. Recent studies at the Mayo Clinic (Johnson, A. et al, 1996) have discounted the prevalent fear of the possible arrhythmogenic effects of imipramine; I, myself, have had NO untoward experiences within this large series. In fact, a cardiologist of my acquaintance is successfully treating some cases of arrhythmia with imipramine!

WARNING: imipramine may cause a significant cross-reaction with Carbocaine or other local anesthetics and it is not advisable to use them together. Either stop the imipramine before the surgical or dental procedure, or use a general anesthetic.

In addition to successfully treating the mis-diagnosed "seriously mentally ill", three more fortuitous implications of this treatment regimen are that a certain number of your cases of alcohol, cocaine, marijuana, caffeine, nicotine, amphetamine (and even some heroin) addiction, those that represent self-medication for this disorder, will be cured; yes, cured! These are the patients who report, "'Speed' allowed me to finish my jobs", or, "Marijuana calmed me down enough to function". Likewise, a certain number of antisocial offenders have their explosive violence or sexual compulsions disappear! We have seen typically drug, domestic violence, or sexual compulsion therapy groups with an incidence of ADD as high as 25-50%! These should be yet other areas of fruitful clinical research.

The fourth targeted population is the successful, high-functioning, surprisingly-often professional group of undiagnosed patients who exhibit perhaps one or two areas of extremely restricted functioning overcome by extra effort in an otherwise superior adaptation. These patients are sometimes readily identified with careful evaluation, but if not, the therapeutic test remains diagnostic. These are the people who perhaps are most rewarded by and rewarding to the practitioner.

This work is dedicated to raising the awareness of both the public and the profession to the fact that this disorder should no longer be viewed as an interesting curiosity of rather minor significance, but rather a major public health issue affecting more people with morbidity and yes, mortality, than many of the traditional public health problems currently delineated, such as the childhood exanthems.

It is likewise dedicated to the multitude of undiagnosed, untreated, or under-treated victims of the disorder whose unnecessary suffering is of such personal and economic magnitude: preventable homicide, suicide, fatal lifestyles, incarceration for life, as well as less dramatic but no less costly lives of severely limited enjoyment and productivity. Having had to defend the patients and myself from the attacks of both the orthodox professionals and the popular press, which has seized upon the controversies to discount the whole concept of the disorder, I have been compelled to become an unapologetic advocate for these patients, which needn't preclude being objective about them.

REFERENCES

Johnson, A., Giuffre, RM, O'Malley, K.(1996): ECG changes in pediatric patients on tricyclic antidepressants, desipramine and imipramine. Can J Psychiatry 41(2):102-6

PROFESSIONAL ADDENDUM
PSYCHODYNAMICS OF A.D.D.

Although most of these by-now almost one thousand patients were seen in short-term settings where there was little opportunity to study them in depth, a few have been in my long-term private practice, and they, along with the multitude of short-term patients, revealed certain commonalities in their personality structure and functioning. How these traits are related to the genetic-organic features of the disorder is not speculated upon here, i.e., causal, consequential, or coincidental, but they are worthy of mention for their own sake.

One gets the distinct impression that the attentional deficit is part of a larger picture of a problem in taking-in in general, through whatever modality, and that this represents a conflict in the oral phase of psychosexual development. The patients seem to be fiercely independent, and largely self-taught and self-feeding. They convey the (implicit) idea that suppliers cannot be entirely relied upon, as exemplified by the poor help they have received so far from the educational and medical establishment. They seem eager but dubious that the new treatment also can be relied upon, often split between a positive transference to the doctor but a negative reaction to the medicine's early side-effects, or other evidence of (pre-)ambivalence.

Many speak about the unreliability and volatility of one or both parents, equally divided between mothers and fathers, with the implicit (envious) deprecation of them as parent figures, even as they are clung to long past adolescence. Since many of the patients are exceptionally bright and creative, one can speculate that they were precocious also, and that there may well have been a disharmony in the parent-infant or -child dialogue, with dissatisfaction, turning passive in-taking into active acquisition, and the development of an envious rivalry toward the parent defending against the warded-off dependency.

One possible scenario is that of the inattentive parent: absent, preoccupied, insensitive or mismatched in sensitivity (intellectual or emotional) to her child, overwhelmed, or afflicted with the inattention disorder herself. Such a parent would not respond to cues of the infant and child in a timely fashion, leading to chronic dissatisfaction, depression, flooding with traumatic overstimulation internally, a steady state of unrelieved tension leading to driven-ness, and paranoid fears of taking-in and being overwhelmed, with possible defenses of avoidance of outside stimuli, seeking of self-satisfaction, premature self-object differentiation (pseudo-separation), premature intellectual development (pseudo-precocity), and an inflated sense of self-importance, denial of dependency, and an envious rivalry with the parent, all rendering an emotional fixation at an infantile level. One can correlate all these phenomena with symptomatic features of the typical case of ADD.

Hypervigilance -> distractibility, insomnia, withdrawal. Precocity -> spurning of parent in false independence, attempt to self-feed and self-learn, focal and thin rather than broad and deep knowledge. Omnipotence -> enhanced self-importance and contempt for parent, society, school -> arguing as if a peer with adults, early drop-out. Feelings of invulnerability -> risk-taking recklessness, sociopathic behavior, experimenting with drugs. Denial of dependence -> addiction potential. Paranoia -> fear of taking in, especially if compelled, and of being overwhelmed with stimuli and emotions (losing internal control) -> need to control the object and relationship with it. Loss of object -> chronic depression, creativity (re-creating that which is lost). Failure to learn, achieve satisfaction -> defeated self-esteem, binging, anorgasmia, early drop-out -> failure to achieve social skills, construct enduring relationships.

Interestingly, many patients after adolescence when they lived at home and attended obligatory school, return to college in their 20's and 30's now on their own and do exceedingly well, although still having to expend extra effort in their studies compared to their classmates. Not a few go from high school drop-outs to straight-A college students, and this before treatment. This occurrence is so common as to support at least a dynamic factor in the disorder, although some would argue it could be a product of maturation alone (which the adult shift to the symptom of body-part movement after childhood total-body hyperkinesis certainly is).

Along with the pseudo-independence is a trait of stubbornness, negativism, or resistance to that which is being told them. They actively do not hear or "pay attention" by turning their minds to other subjects, forgetting, or not taking-in in the first place. They can be made to pay heed by special attention warnings ala the U.S.Navy's, "Now hear this!", or when they themselves are interested in a study of their own choosing, on which they are able to lavish hours of uninterrupted concentration (and ignoring of all else). This perhaps is the revealing clue to the psychodynamics of the patient, feeding himself with something which interests (and temporarily satisfies) his quick mind, while spurning the efforts of parents and teachers to do the same, denying them satisfaction and thereby making himself altogether a "handful" to manage as student or child.

Along with this conflict on the dependency-independency axis, with its roots in the oral and early anal phases, is the related issue of mistrust, of people and of what they have to offer. Not only are the patients poor listeners and readers but picky eaters, and have a problem therefore in obtaining satisfaction. Not only offerings from others but their own productions often fail to satisfy, accounting for the tendency to not finish projects and to seek anew to find satisfaction elsewhere. Here we see both paranoia preventing in-taking, and envy spoiling that which has been sampled. The natural resultant of the strong needs and equally strong defenses against satisfaction results in a steady-state of frustration, with its attendant rise in intrapsychic tension. This then seeks discharge or relief in the many modes already covered: muscular tension, driven-ness (pseudo-mania), emotional volatility and outbursts, sedation through stimulation-seeking (self-controlled excitement) and novelty-attraction, and most significantly, the seeking of surcease through an attachment to a self-administered agent (addiction). Reading of novels (prepared phantasy), hobbies, physical workouts and sports, sexuality, and substance use are among the popular activities to which they may become habituated.

The patient is struggling with his unmet needs to be fed (reliably), his suspicion that he will not be, his wish that he could take care of his own needs in superior fashion to the methods of the parent, his awareness that he can neither satisfy himself nor allow himself to be satisfied, his yearning to put his superior intelligence to some productive (and hence satisfying) use but his apparent inability to do so, and/or even to understand himself or be understood by others. This hopeless circle is what leads to moods of suicidal despondency.

In technical terms, he is manifesting a manic defense against dependency and merger anxiety (loss of self: paranoia) in the regressive direction, separation anxiety (depression) in the progressive direction, fixated on the horns of a dilemma in an enduring narcissistic state I have labeled as borderline in previous writings. This is a very stable configuration which resists major therapeutic intervention, though it can benefit from spaced, long-term reliable therapeutic relationships (small bites, unforced, enduring), but which is always subject to the narcissist's tendency to relinquish his objects, the negative therapeutic reaction, or temporary regressions in functioning, sometimes to a psychotic level.

The source of the chief unconscious resistance to treatment of such a patient is the threat of loss of control of the treatment situation, which he has usually successfully manipulated thus far (with the feared development of true transference: falling under the influence). These patients have a typical need to possess and control their objects in an infantile mode of (defense against an) object-relationship, a product of early anal fixation. Tellingly, when they have achieved total mastery of their object, as in a pupil achieving special educational measures and especially one-on-one tutoring, or when they function as their own tutor, they are able to take-in and learn without difficulty! This, of course, testifies to the dynamic nature of their inattention, and would seem to augur well for the possibility of psychotherapy, although their resistance renders them prone to grasp the tutor/therapist and keep him at arm's length throughout the encounter.

A.D.D.: Professional Addendum Psychodynamics Of A.D.D.

It is no wonder that he is often mis-diagnosed as manic-depressive, depressive, or paranoid, for he has these features to be sure; however, they do not encompass nor characterize the total clinical picture, merely reflecting symptomatic elements of it. When his symptoms are unusually severe resulting in illiteracy, gross inarticulateness, and disorganization of thinking, he can be easily mistaken for a patient with mental retardation or florid psychosis. Probably the appropriate descriptive diagnosis for many ADD sufferers with a fixed character disorder is Borderline or Narcissistic Personality Disorder; but, to be remembered, not all ADDers have a character disorder along with it.

A PSYCHOANALYST LOOKS AT ALCOHOLICS ANONYMOUS (ADDENDUM IV)

I have recently had the opportunity to study a so-called chemical dependency in-patient unit (so named in the East, more often and more accurately substance abuse in the West), run along the lines of AA by a team of mental health workers of mixed backgrounds led by alcohol counselors (often recovered users themselves), with the nominal inclusion of a psychiatric member for necessary codifying and prescribing functions, but more for legitimizing and marketing purposes than genuine collaboration, I fear. The experience was illuminating in several respects, particularly related to the themes in this paper.

First of all, the patient population was almost exclusively Catholic, predominantly Irish, some Italian , with rare Protestant and Jewish patients. The composition of the staff was unknown to me, but seemed consistent with the indigenous general population of friendly but moralistic, parsimonious New England Yankees. The philosophy of the program administered, directly drawn from AA, was nominally non-sectarian religious with overtones of both Christian divisions: an undisguised authoritarianism ("We know best", "You will do this now"), and a similarly undisguised public Evangelism with group confessions of having fallen, guilt, and personal powerlessness (and thus responsibility-lessness, and thus demonization of the liquor "bug"), an appeal to the Lord for help, an appeal to the group for support, and a process of purification which bordered on exorcism of the inhabiting devil...all covered over with a pseudo-scientific patina of "disease", which the medical profession, I fear, has too readily uncritically bought into.

Although there is a superficially open acceptance of anyone who desires to join the AA program, it is uncritical and anonymous (contained in the name of the organization and its practice: "No last names, please"). In addition and more importantly, the acceptance is highly conditional on identifying with the program, and thus experienced as partial at best. Along with the various strictures and prohibitions placed upon the individual, he would not be too far off to experience the acceptance as actual rejection with a thin gloss of "treatment" ("for your own good").

And actually, this is what the vast majority of the patients experienced in their home environment, being overtly thrown out of their homes for substance abuse, after having been covertly rejected out of, I believe, a cold nature in their partners or a parallel dependency there which likewise limited the support they were able to give. This seemed to be the most frequent theme in the histories. Many of the patients described spouses who seemed unable to love, too needy themselves, narcissistically self-involved, or described as "saints" (for their patient enduring of the patient's misbehavior) while the patient readily accepted the total blame for their own "sinning" . Most of the patients came to treatment in the midst of physical separation, divorce, or court-ordered injunctions to stay away from the family. These patients (and not a few of their separated spouses!) were pathetically eager for a warm and accepting therapeutic relationship with a psychiatrist and worked very well and rapidly in it, demonstrating thereby a high degree of psychological-mindedness, insight, and capacity for object-relations as well as their deprivation of it. However, this good relationship was perceived by the staff as antithetical to the purposes of the program (as was any socialization or fraternization of the patients with each other) and was either covertly sabotaged or overtly countermanded.

Second in frequency was the theme of quite conscious identification by the men with their (dead) father's drinking (and their shared rejection by the mother), often down to the pattern of the drinking, behavior while intoxicated, and even the brand of liquor consumed; the women complained of un-loving husbands, displaced from earlier histories with their mothers. Next in frequency was the theme of intervention of the authorities because of criminal behavior while under the influence or in dealing narcotics (acting "bad"), with it's corresponding (or causative) sense of guilt and ready acceptance of the punitive environment (to be sure, less so than jail time, although a surprising number opted for the latter given the alternative of a "therapeutic" disposition).

A Psychoanalyst Looks At Alcoholics Anonymous (Addendum IV)

Equally frequent was the history of physical and/or sexual abuse in childhood, but because of its recent media popularization and the consequent hypersensitivity to the possibility among the patient population and staff alike (who also express the clinical wisdom that this finding is frequent among substance abusers), its real frequency ought to be more carefully studied, as would befit all of these etiologic factors.

There was a smaller sub-group of patients, a residual category if you will, that did not seem to share the psychodynamic characteristics of the others, consisting of apparent "losers" or people with inadequate personalities who had turned to drugs and crime as part of their social mal-adaptation, and who did not seem influence-able by any rehabilitation efforts, becoming recurrent relapsers and upon whom repeated efforts seemed wasted (not to deter the business of rehabilitation, however).

The related observation was the high rate of relapse and recidivism in the total patient population, and the staff's and administration's apparent ready tolerance of it, rationalized as just an expected normal aspect of the "disease". I could not escape the impression that there was an unconscious encouragement of relapse, effected by undue shortening of the "therapeutic" experience (rationalized as economic necessity, which was belied by the multiplied cost of repeated treatments, which suggests in turn the possibility of a more venal motive), and the encouragement of a regressive dependent relationship with the authoritarian power structure of the organization, which dependence was merely endured and ultimately discouraged out of simple fatigue and in the name of weaning. (This in contradistinction to our psychiatric use of regression as a means to the re-educative goal of achievement of genuine autonomy.)

I came away from the experience frustrated by the blocking of my therapeutic efforts and clinical expertise, and angry by the rebuff experienced at the hands of denying "helpers", but reconfirmed in my conviction that alcoholism and drug abuse are oral deficiency syndromes, a product of an attempted relationship with a non-nurturing object, with the abuse a symptom only, a seductive habit to be sure, the so-called "physiological dependence" a factual but thin, non-operative factor (many users give up their "habits" readily and repeatedly when conditions change: e.g. soldiers' un-hooking from heroin post-Vietnam).

This is not to say that for a certain sub-population of alcoholics, the AA approach is not a pragmatic and semi-successful attempt to deal with an overwhelming public health problem in our society. But we must be careful not to over-generalize this acknowledgement into a prescription for all our patients, particularly intelligent, educated, and relationship-able ones who can be and are helped by psychotherapy and psychoanalysis much more enduringly every day of the week in our practices. And we should be careful about our scientific conceptualizations of this syndrome: that should remain pure.

Freud himself spoke of the necessity of alloying psychoanalysis in the treatment of problems of everyday life, and this institutional approach to this clinical syndrome may be just such an example. However, the ringing in of Psychiatry by AA in hospital units variously described as "Dual-Focus", "Dual-Diagnosis", and "Dual-Track" may be less a synergistic collaboration than an uncomplimentary exploitation of us.

"AS-IF" PERSONALITY: A CLINICAL CAUTION

June 17, 2010

In 1934, Dr. Helene Deutsch first described unanalyzable patients who appear treatable but fail to engage in the therapeutic process. She described the subjects as appearing perfectly normal but somehow inauthentic, aping behavior from their environment, acting rather than being. You can familiarize yourself with her original description by Googling the title, which won't be repeated here.

She offered no dynamic explanation in this brief introduction, though a colleague Dr. Masud Kahn proposed a super-ego defect and she wondered if there was an underlying schizoid syndrome. Having attempted to analyze two patients resembling her description, I believe I have uncovered a dynamic operative in those cases.

Ignatius X, a twenty-ish single artist was employed in color work, while painting was his hobby. Why he came for help I cannot recall, but he seemed genuinely motivated to cooperate in a 5-time/week classical analysis. This was pursued by an eager young candidate with furor therapeuticus, alas, to no avail.

He associated (and I interpreted) according to the recipe, and was perfectly satisfied to go on endlessly, although the interpreter came to realize that he, himself, was not, for in total agreement with Deutsch realized nothing was happening as treatment wore on. No insights, no change in behavior, no discoveries, no deepening, no development, and no dissatisfaction with that state of affairs.

To amplify, he belonged to a normal-appearing social circle, one member of which knew me and referred him. I don't think he was regarded as odd in this circle, i.e. was socially adept. Two features of his functioning remain in my memory: his artistic prints were colorful, elaborate architectural constructions absolutely devoid of life, warmth, symbolic content, or evoking of emotion in the viewer. And the second, his favorite language noun was "form", modified by another describing the type of form, e.g. life-form, circle-form, building-form, etc. These were not actual entities in reality, but representations of them. Deutsch does posit "A lack of cathexis in their objects" in these patients.

Realizing my interventions were having no effect whilst he continued to offer me material to elicit my interest, I determined that his aim was exactly that, to keep me interested. He was, by so doing, keeping me and holding me closer. This, I believe, is the functioning dynamic at work, controlling the analyst as the young infant holds and controls his mother. It is the seeking and preservation of intimacy of a primordial kind, the achievement of which afforded him all the satisfaction he sought.

The young analyst, frustrated at his seemingly meaningless efforts, stopped responding to his patient's presented clues and so tried silence as a therapeutic technique. Five weeks went by with absolutely no change in his behavior, and so, when he realized he lost control of me, he left. No regrets, no recriminations, no emotion of any kind. I am not especially delighted with my experiment, but at least I now feel I understand it. But I do have regrets at not having helped him.

The posited "lack of cathexis of their objects" means their "significant others" are not real to them, not incorporated object representations with feelings and meaning attached, not residua of actual historical relationships but "forms" of them, as the patient would say This incorporation of abiding internal objects normally ensues from meaningful relationships with separate real people, a phase following the primitive controlling/merging relationship with mother which the patient is trying to recapture, and typically is enhanced with the loss of the real relationship (as separating and moving beyond).

This "as-if" symptomatology suggests the original relationship with mother was never successfully achieved and graduated from. The possible

"As-If" Personality: A Clinical Caution

whys are manifold: early loss of her, inability of her's to bond with her infant or to wean him from it once established, some unknown limitation of his, who knows? So the individual physically grows up acting with unreal representations of real people, acting inauthentic himself, a poseur so to speak.

Whether free associations from the couch, or the conversations from the chair, both seem real enough as the therapist tries to empathize with what is being communicated so as to understand it and respond. But the talk is not shared communication but vocal acts, serving as provocation of the therapist's reactions, primary process we call it. Not only are people not real to him, but words likewise are not, often merely aping of what the therapist said. It is certainly possible that gradations of these qualities can be found in different individuals, more or less so to speak, but the underlying meaninglessness is unmistakable and arouses a counter-transference reaction in the therapist of at first boredom, then frustration, then resentment at being fooled.

What about subjects that adopt acting as a profession, can they be successfully analyzed? They give a typical history of dropping out of high school to join the stage, possibly a clue to their educability and use of manipulation of their audience; years of attempts with them have left me no clear answer. Other narcissistic personalities of divers stripes, gypsies, con-artists, other dissimulators are likewise problematic. The British Object-Relations School of Melanie Klein, Winnicott, et al addresses these early stages of functioning utilizing such concepts as symbiosis, projective identification, false self and others claim possible therapeutic effect; of this I cannot attest.

On a superficial level, these subjects could be seen as a caricature of adolescents making trial identifications of admired models before consolidating into an organized identity (and growing up)...hence may benefit more from a mentor (coach) than psychiatric "therapy". The analyst, sensing this patient's actual need and responding to his/her typical seductiveness may find himself abandoning his "blank screen" and offering himself as a real object, yet another countertransference hazard.

Far from a problematic analytic lapse, however, the recognition of the role of the "real" therapist has given rise to a whole school of theory and technique by Bettleheim in Chicago called "The Corrective Emotional Experience", and in Los Angeles and New York by men like Greenson, arguing the therapeutic value of the real relationship vs. the transference one.

"THE BOOTSTRAPPERS": A CONTEMPORARY CHARACTEROLOGY.

William S. Horowitz, M.D.

This discussion will endeavor to describe common patients in my practice who are the adult product of the under-parented child, who as a consequence feel they have raised themselves: hence the title. They seek out assistance for a variety of nominal problems but shortly reveal themselves to be feeling stalled and bored with their repetitive life going nowhere, a product of a character disorder of life-long duration (plus the possibility of organic change) entailing particular resistances and challenges in the treatment.

I

They present as narcissistic or borderline characters who essentially lead an isolated life whether or not amongst others; who are usually strikingly successful in their chosen vocation by virtue of their intelligence, boldness, exploitativeness, charm, manipulativeness, intense envy-driven competitiveness, recklessness, cynicism, and lack of social constraints; who feel never-the-less goal-less and unfulfilled, isolated and alienated from others, depressed and paranoid; overtly desirous of intimate human relations but puzzlingly unable to consummate them, and envious of the normals who can; unreceptive and un-dependent, self-taught and uneducated; taking what they want from life and blaming others and conditions; feeling simultaneously powerful and helpless, superior and inferior, unusually intelligent but ignorant of their problem, advantaged and disadvantaged, and unaffiliated; and with thoughts of death never far in the background.

These are men usually but not exclusively, who either marry early, late, or never, but throughout have the psychology of the confirmed bachelor. I.e., considering themselves exceptions to the social pattern, they feel unobligated to their birth families and their society, unobligated and not dependent on their wives or girlfriends either, feeling instead that they are owed something and being exceptional have the right to take what they fancy. They look upon their married brethren as "suckers" who have fallen for the social trap, while their own existence is infinitely more efficient. They are un-domesticated, like perpetual juvenile males in animal groups who hang around together and take no part in family life, never growing up. As this would suggest, they are highly narcissistic and covertly homosexual.

Their worst conscious fear is to be a sucker themselves, to "fall for" a girl, or a therapist and his therapy; their worst preconscious fear is then to be abandoned, again. Paralleling these social fears is the frequent symptom of a fear of swimming, letting go of the side of the pool, immersing, submersing, and/or being inundated by waves, all representing the self-withholding, narcissistic defense against the deeply repressed fear/wish for involvement (to be "in the swim") and ultimately fusion.

They uniformly give the history of a lack of parenting, either through: (1) early loss of parent(s); (2) absence of parenting models in their parents' experience (a parent who was a bootstrapper herself – two had mothers raised in an orphanage); (3) parental immaturity (maternal narcissism) or neurotic conflict about parenting (paternal distancing from their daughters and sons out of sexual anxiety); (4) consummated incest; (5) Significant disparity between the generations' intellectual or cultural levels or age, which served to weaken the parenting experience; (6) undermining of parental authority by grandparents, other spouse, or the courts in the not infrequent case of divorce; (7) significant parental dependency which encourages a premature reversal of generations; and (8) operations within the child, such as competitiveness, adolescent rebellion, sexual anxiety, and particularly premature disillusionment, which serve to distance the child from the parents and undermine their influence.

All left home early, many after a history of home or school adjustment failure, complaining that they had missed their childhood; from here they

"The Bootstrappers": A Contemporary Characterology

may affiliate with another family, begin their own with early marriage and children, or develop an "institutional transference" to a school, military, business, club, gang of similarly situated, or a career of psychotherapy. They either do not know or refuse to observe common social convention, their lack of habit training (work, study, language, hygiene, diet, manners, etc.) testifying to the absence of or defiance against effective parenting, particularly mothering, making the analyst wonder if they were "raised in a barn".

He might, e.g.,: neglect to brush his teeth; habitually belch or fart or yawn in company, blow his nose into his napkin at table or pick it there; avoid writing letters, print in all capital letters, or misuse personal pronouns; not close the door after himself; wear tennis shoes and short pants to all occasions, etc.

They are attracted to treatment by loneliness and the hope for (parasitic) object replacement and implicitly by the undemanding narcissistic gratification offered, but are drawn into the most exquisite contention with the parent surrogate to whom they have never successfully related.

One early memory dated to the age of three concerns criticizing her mother's preparations in the kitchen, in time getting her to retire in tears... antedating a life-long pattern of harassing her coaches, professors, employers, and husbands with her superior knowledge of their trade, looking to defeat them, which, more often than not, she did.

What ensues is a battle with the parental object similar to the earliest phase of secondary narcissism, the "terrible twos", however with all the success and power the adult-patient has accumulated compared to the helpless (?) child. The new analyst-parent seems destined to lose the power struggle, as did indeed the actual parents and their first surrogates, the maid and teacher. Besides arguing their superior knowledge of their own functioning and what they need from the analyst, they will attempt to compete with him in all other imagined arenas.

Scheduling lengthy business trips abroad, adopting children secretly, buying multiple homes or expensive tax-shelters, marrying or divorcing abruptly, etc., can all have competitive implications toward the analyst's private activities or therapeutic endeavors with the patient.

As with other narcissistic characters, they exhibit the three "P's": pretension (infantile grandiosity and magical identification), presumption (lack of firm ego boundaries and object-representations), and provocation (manipulating the object to control it)[1]. These infantile qualities, the three P's, lend themselves to a proclivity to acting, to believing that by pretending that they are somebody they become that somebody, the basis for the "as-if" quality in the eponymous character first described by Deutsch (1942)[2]. An appreciation of this quality in these patients is essential to not being taken in by them, and the coming to grips with the actual transactions taking place in their object-relationships which is necessary for therapeutic progress.

Many took their envy-driven competitiveness onto the sports field and actually excelled there (to state championship level) as they later do in business or professional life. Most but not all of my series are men, and their presenting battles are with father-figures, accompanied by the unabashed conscious idea they were their own fathers to themselves. Their actual fathers were distant (aloof, working long hours), ill, or absent (sailors, traveling salesmen, or divorced). In several cases, the fathers were present but their work involved secrecy, rendering themselves and what they did unavailable to the son.

But these battles are usually a recap of an inability to form a trusting, dependent, antecedent relationship with the mother, who early on becomes bossed by the precocious son. Further, some give the history of an even earlier "honeymoon" period with mother and/or her female relatives, with a pronounced period of infantile grandiosity which they were later unable to relinquish and subordinate to a dependent relationship within the family.

The ordinal position within the family did not seem significant. A few were only or middle children, most either first or last-born.

Their sudden dethronement after the birth of a younger sibling, in several cases, aroused sustained bruising hostility in the older toward the healthier rival, acted-out by brutalizing his sib's trusting idealization of him. Their former exceptional status now lost, reinforced by the circumstance of primogeniture, both combined to inflate their infantile demandingness for redress to an unmodifiable extent and render them untreatable narcissistic personality disorders.

Some of the younger patients, on the other hand, had a near "twinship" relationship with their next oldest sib, who, when similarly disturbed, colluded with and compounded the delinquent personality disorder in both. Whether the identified patient is the older or younger sib, however, an emotional clinging in their loneliness could be seen between the two closest sibs.

Many of the families had long ago felt defeated and relinquished parental authority and caretaking to a hired maid, usually an uneducated Negro in my series, and the patients exhibit a profound learning disability which seems to be in part an early reaction to and identification with her; the major psychodynamic contribution, however, I believe comes from both an early defiant feeding disturbance and its related premature ego development in these patients which produces a variety of experimental, ad hoc, fragmented self-teaching rather than a trusting coherently-organized incorporated learning from the teacher[3].

But in addition to this dynamic, a good many of the patients seem to exhibit what has been described in the descriptive psychiatric literature as a borderline organicity or M(inimal) B(rain) D(ysfunction), with one or several of the symptoms enumerated below predominating. There was only one patient with a definitive history of head injury with personality change, though many were active in sports. Almost all had a poor diet filled with junk foods (self-feeders); two patients were probably hyperkinetic in childhood, and these two became addicted to the self-administration of stimulant drugs in adulthood. Various theories have been expounded for this syndrome of Attention Deficit Disorder, one of the older ones being dietary[4], one of the newer ones being hypertestosteroneism. The etiology is otherwise unknown.

Symptoms include: 1) a symbolic or abstracting impairment which may be manifested by the learning disorder above, a variety of receptive or expressive dyslexia[5], or an object(person)-naming deficiency; 2) difficulty in pattern recognition, particularly noticeable in geographic (traffic) or social disorientation, getting lost or not "getting the picture", thus being unable to fit themselves into the mis-perceived social situation; 3) difficulty remembering what has been told them or what they have told you already; 4) an attention deficit, with poor concentration and retention (they have an inordinate difficulty in sustaining attention to a lecture or performance or your interventions without drawing attention to themselves).

5) An affective flattening, dullness, or constriction, a product of overcontrol because of the feared tendency to lability and explosive outbursts, or a sustained mood of excitement barely controlled; 6) constricted (pseudo-phobic), driven (pseudo-manic), counter-phobic, impulsive, anti-social, or erratic behavior.

Symptoms 5 & 6 may be a product not only of stimulating drugs, but the proclivity to self-stimulation in general, represented by masturbation and risky behavior, perhaps a product of (a) the subject's discovery earlier in life of the paradoxical sedative or controlling effect of (the discharge of) excitement, (b) poor emotional control, and (c) the dynamic avoidance of boredom and the passive state.

7) A tendency to confusional episodes; 8) pseudo-relationships which lack a true bilaterality or perception of the other as a person like himself, resembling more the parallel play of children; 9) difficulty planning, organizing, and executing tasks and intentions, with babyish lapses, sometimes pleading to be led but then having difficulty following even simple direction; 10) a susceptibility to being overwhelmed with stimuli (catastrophic reaction), new experience, or challenges to their (defective) understanding, with a resultant avoidance of learning situations

"The Bootstrappers": A Contemporary Characterology

and the external world, rendering altogether a rigid, no growth, (agora-) phobic, or coarcted personality; and 11) perceptual-motor uncoordination such as strabismus and clumsiness, or sub-clinical choreo-athetoid movements.

To balance the clinical picture, many of them have compensating skills which are truly impressive and are used to mask their deficiencies; altogether, the degree of their impairment is variable, and may not be at all noticeable in the therapy situation, only to become glaringly apparent in social settings or their writing.

To compound the conceptual dilemma, many if not all of these symptoms could be explained in psychodynamic or functional terms. For instance, the learning disorder can be viewed as a product of a rebellious and paranoid refusal to take in, the inattention as narcissistic concentration on the self and "not giving a shit" about the external world, the disorientation from not knowing their place, deficient psychomotor control from poor habit training from defiance (incontinence), etc. The issue remains an open one in my mind, though I have seen dramatic diminution and even disappearance of selected symptoms in different cases, inclining me toward a functional explanation. On the other hand, some symptoms respond quite nicely to medication.

The women (and younger siblings) in their lives are passive, compliant, and profoundly inadequate-feeling (defeated), after incessant attacks on their adequacy under the guise of pseudo-parenting which masks the patient's profound breast envy. Marital and other relationships are also pseudo-, in that the partner is captivated into the relationship by induced (projected and manipulated) dependence on the subject, while he has what he needs without acknowledgement of that need; i.e., he continues the illusion of independence while seducing all into needing him[6].

The frequency of the term "pseudo" in this description correlates with the "as-if" or acting nature of their behavior mentioned earlier.

This is the background which allows him to continue his deprecating attacks on the neediness of his object while he enacts the role of parent, meanwhile feeding on the parasitized object-libido or care (-taking) of his partner. He sucks the good out of her, discharges his effluvia into her, feels renewed at her expense, and leaves her feeling drained, worthless, and toxic.

In the defense against the transference, he phantasizes or attempts to prove that the analyst needs his supplies (fees and patienthood) and that is what guarantees the treatment compact, though he may give lip service to all the "help" the analyst has provided, chiefly to seduce his continued interest. After having established in his own mind the unevenness of the relationship, he feels free to absent himself for short or even long periods because of all he has done for the analyst, and his need for relief of the burden of it. (See below the pivotal importance of "recesses", which, if not arranged, may be forced.)

But there is another dynamism at work here. The patient perceived the parent as narcissistic, more interested in herself than her child, and it is this perceived narcissism of the object, not entirely the product of his own incomplete separation of self from her, which is being attacked. The patient is very wary of crediting or needing such a narcissistic person for fear of feeding that very overestimation of her importance and of handing over that power to her to emotionally capture him. The attack tends to become generalized into devaluing everything she has to offer, attacking both her (and his own) narcissism and her realistic self-value and -esteem, rendering her useless and unattractive to him. In the process, everybody's self-esteem including the patient's is minimized, in an orgy of asceticism, disillusionment, and humiliating self-abnegation.

A successful businessman might boast that everything he owned in the world could be fitted into the back seat of his car, or a successful professional might enter analysis owning one pair of shoes. Related to this is the symptom of inability to enjoy a good night's sleep, making a virtue of how little sleep he required. A similar pattern governed eating, picking up minimal snacks on the run while scoffing at others' neediness and self-indulgence.

II

The struggle between objects immediately alerts us to the structural situation: this is a pre-transference phenomenon, before complete self-object separation has taken place (in fact it is the process of effecting that self-object separation), before abiding object-representations have been established, before internalization of defense has taken place, before a time sense is in place which would permit displacement from past to current objects (transference proper). It has been called the "false" transference. 1

Part-self and part-object representations are intermingled in a purified-pleasure or parasitic arrangement with incorporation of the good and expulsion of the bad, so-called "projective" and magical identification, idealization, isolation and splitting (or lack of integration), and externalization (or lack of internalization) and controlling of the object are prominent. (Have you noticed also that all these early narcissistic defenses begin with the letter "I"?)

The patient is not struggling between impulse and internal defense, but with his object, attempting to establish his own self at the expense of his object. Dynamically, the patient is caught on the horns of a dilemma, between merger/paranoia in the regressive direction and separation/depression in the progressive, manifesting the manic (narcissistic/parasitic) defense. Thus is the state of affairs with object-relations, which are characterized by aggression toward the object.

As far as the classical stages of libidinal development are concerned, they are exhibited in manifold ways but are essentially unintegrated or split off from the correlated stages of object-relations. Oral manifestations have to do with denials, projections and reaction-formations against the underlying urges to touch, suck, merge, sleep, dream, dissolve, be swallowed up, etc.

These patients may be loudly or quietly demanding, domineering and manipulative, being used to running everything; picky poor eaters who are fond of junk food; anorectic, bulimic, and/or addicted; picky poor readers fond of junk readings; poor sleepers; "touchy", distancing, and paranoid; argumentative poor students who have a good intelligence but are pseudo-stupid and uneducated (from a very real learning disturbance); have high unsatisfiable expectations, being perfectionistic, idealistic and greedy; feel invulnerable, magically powerful, and not yet susceptible to the passage of time; or in another form of oceanic fusion may be naive, innocent, and gullible, a "nature child".

In some, a later anal struggle with the object is prominent: they are contentious and stubborn; constipated, speech and urine-retentive; lacking personal hygiene and social manners, or have elaborate reaction-formations against the soiling impulse (in the women displaced to the nose which chronically runs and is not blown); susceptible to muscular spasms; experience sadistic controlling and torturing phantasies and actions; live out a masochistic, pleasureless existence whether in a life-style of self-indulgence, asceticism, or a paradoxical mixture of the two; have an early history of enemas and whippings and later cruelty to their younger siblings and partners; have few if any children themselves (un-fecund) and make poor parents; are imitative rather than creative; and disagreeable, ungiving and unpleasant.

In yet others, phallic-level derivatives seem to dominate the clinical picture. They manifest an intense competitiveness in their business or profession and sports as well as human relationships in general; are unusually aggressive and litigious[7]; intolerant of being ignored, their appearance is of great importance to them (many of the men had cosmetic surgery, by the mother in childhood or themselves in adulthood); likewise is their and their women's slimness fanatically valued, representing not only phallic

"The Bootstrappers": A Contemporary Characterology

qualities but the absence of femininity, breasts, neediness, self-indulgence, and having something to offer.

When of short stature they are inclined to erect themselves to their full height and strut (colloquially known as having "Little Man's Disease"); enjoy the use of machines, tools, weapons and vehicles; have phantasies of penetrating sadistic attacks on females, particularly their breasts; can exhibit a machine-like undistracted concentration on tasks and ram them through to completion (in addition to being mechanically inclined, several had the unconscious phantasy that they were machines); and altogether project an unemotional jock image (which may not include having a girl-friend).

Needless to emphasize, they are selfish, arrogant, and disrespectful of or oblivious to others as persons too, only objects to be guarded against or exploited ("need-satisfying"; is this perhaps the origin of the term instinctual "object"?). In their social relations, when not observing from the sidelines, they tend to be controlling, overbearing, and intimidating, bulldozing their way over and around others to get their way. When thwarted, stood up to, or merely confronted with the general expectations held of others, they tend toward reactions of indignation over their unrecognized specialness (the "Prince/Princess" phenomenon).

Their lack of a firm identity plus their refusal to subordinate themselves in their family nexus renders them not "knowing their place", which combines with the social disorientation mentioned earlier to render them either avoiding of social intercourse altogether or clumsily attempting to fit in; needless to say, they resist being put in their place, or accepting any limits that they themselves do not impose. In many, their magical identifications and pretensions render them "phony" which also "turns off" potential object-relationships. Asleep and awake, they tend to turn their back on others.

These varieties of pre-genital character demonstrate that these narcissistic traits are not limited to just the historically-identified phallic-narcissistic type, but exist at all libidinal levels; what they have in common is a narcissistic fixation in their object-relations.

Many are preoccupied with their bodily appearance and processes and are fearful of disease; hypochondriasis is part of their narcissistic libidinal configuration: one can observe this preoccupation waning as the interest in external objects grows. Masturbation is prominent and preferred. The masturbatory phantasy, which is often acted-out outside but unreported to the analyst before eventually being acted-out within the treatment itself, is that of lying on his back and being masturbated or fellated, which may well have been an infantile experience (a not unheard of practice among uneducated baby-sitters); or of being enemized, which is regularly remembered and feared/wished for in the transference (as a manipulative ploy toward the analyst). Pets, plants, and toys play an especially important role as transitional objects for these lonely people, and books and films are vicarious lives.

In the case of the absent father, an unreal phantasied super-ego and/or ego-ideal father-figure is constructed, who, under the influence of primitive idealization is perfectionistic, demanding, dominating and oppressing the subject into self-abnegation and pleasurelessness. This paternal conscience/ideal, like the phallic masculine identification described above, is a caricature of manliness, and testifies to the absence of an actual male model and/or the superordination of a female identification.

The patient's claim that he was father to himself reflects at least a psychological truth in that he has a dual identity as both father and son, one of several dichotomies or splits in his structure. Under the influence of the real analyst, these ego structures are modifiable into more integrated, realistic, potent, loving and forgiving ones.

Needless to add, the cases are not uniform and display unique admixtures depending on quality and duration of parenting experience at home, later intercurrent life experience (which may include organic injury), and genetic endowment[8]. In addition to the above, neurotic conflicts are

"The Bootstrappers": A Contemporary Characterology

present (typically obsessional in the men and hysterical in the women), as well as suppressed grandiose delusions, all of which require their appropriate handling.

As children they commonly had the experience of being left to look after themselves if not younger siblings. Some with latch-keys in their pockets, they were miniature adults as children. With the physical and/or emotional absence of their parent, they felt on their own, a striking stance they bring into the treatment situation as well as new social relationships: they evidence a unilaterality or one-wayness in their consideration of intercourse with others. And, from this early "escape" or "release" from the family nexus, they no longer feel as participants but rather observers of the scene, a position they carry into their adult Weltanschauung. This accounts for the alienation and unaffiliation they feel with others and social institutions.

I have had the opportunity to observe, not treat, a sibling pair whose mother left the home to work when the younger started school, the minimal mothering function thereafter being provided by father whose employment brought him home early, often to cook. The younger female sib, who recalls that she stayed after school until supper-time from an early age on, had a precocious and brilliant academic and athletic career until her classic schizophrenic break in college, possibly precipitated by the cumulative loss of her two-year older brother to college, her deeply-beloved betrothed, and her "motherland" on an extended trip abroad.

The acute illness was succeeded by chronic active disease controlled by medication and a loose obsessional defense which permitted her finishing two advanced degrees, after which her behavioral adjustment settled at a self-sustaining but childishly regressed level, being entirely comfortable and satisfied with a protected perfunctory job at her former university department! (family). Her style of living was simple, and her main libidinal interests were eating, doing her jobs, and counting her small savings account.

Her two-year older brother became a somewhat aggressive personality disorder with prominent oral interests, maintaining a marginal social, occupational and artistic career adjustment. The striking feature of both now-adults was their acted-out passive dependency impulses and motherless-hallmark uncouthness in the presence of unusual intelligence and artistic talent. Both reportedly had been drug users in their youth. The "control", so to speak, was an older first-born brother who had 4-6 more years respectively of mothering, who attained a superior social, heterosexual, vocational, artistic and intellectual level of achievement, and became married with children and a leader in his social and academic community.

The unprotected, insecure child coping on his own in a frightening world of possibilities is above all else anxious: this leads to a bravado and false sense of power (omnipotence), which in turn inevitably provokes control from the outside. Feared situations are avoided or brazenly explored. In addition, impulses arising internally are attempted to be controlled by means of undoing (often ritualized) acts giving rise to compulsions; and/or isolated thoughts are attacked with counter-thoughts leading to obsessions. What results is a mixed picture of impulse-ridden delinquency combined with failing obsessive-compulsive defenses, phobic avoidances and counter-phobic actions, and the experimenting with drugs to control the anxiety-ridden state.

Only slightly less prominent is the underlying sense of abandonment and futility, the depression, which mitigates against trying. We could say the bootstrapper is suffering from a chronic anxious depression masked by a narcissistic character. His precocious pseudo-maturity overlaying his obvious childishness could be thought of as psychological progeria, which conveys the very real morbidity of the disorder.

Parenthetically, these children are not all from poor families; most had highly successful mothers and fathers, who, however, forwent their parenting roles for one reason or another (in the case of too-busy-for-treatment patients, it is easy to see what their parental model was: often two working parents). And substituting a Negro mammy or even healthy step-parent

"The Bootstrappers": A Contemporary Characterology

who fed and loved the child rarely contributed significant parental authority. These are the "street children" from our own side of the tracks.

They scrutinize the analyst's and their own functioning in exquisite detail, having the utmost difficulty in allowing the separate functional roles of patient and analyst, wanting to be the analyst themselves. Their observations about you are used for manipulative, controlling purposes; about themselves as self-analysis.

Often they will start the hour with a casual observation about how you seem to be feeling today, attempting thereby to put you on the defensive and to seize control of the hour from the very beginning. Other manifestations of the controlling urge are manifold: impatience about being kept waiting to start, watching the clock and ending the hour themselves, starting off with a barrage of material designed to put you off and even out, speaking overly loudly (long-distance, non-intimate), and speaking dramatically as if a performance for effect on an unseen audience. The content is thus not the issue, but the manner of delivery which carries out the instinctual aims: "the medium is the message".

As for learning, they argue. (One actually went on to become a lawyer, all were legalistic and litigating.) Resisting the analyst's insights and interpretations, they insist on offering their own superior versions (not all worthless by any means) to instruct the instructor, or offer him criticism from their own accumulated experience with previous unsuccessful therapies, ala a supervisor.

Rarely they also read about treatment, but that is the exception for the habit of study and learning even from books is eschewed, so that they are poor scholars and essentially uneducated (by no means incompatible with being a successful professional). Chiefly it is their own idiosyncratic ideas which they wish to promulgate and have validated. They are therefore socially parochial.

A patient might pointedly never pick up the magazines in the waiting room but on occasion bring his own business papers for perusal, which might raise the question in the analyst's mind of whether he was masking functional illiteracy.

Many will volunteer the role- or generation-reversal or peerage which existed early on in certain family functions, but be unaware of the ubiquity and inappropriateness of his attitude in current life. Closer inspection reveals a long history of such power struggles between patient and parent (-surrogate), reflecting the little big one's omnipotent and grandiose, paranoid, un-depending, envious and competitive relation with the parent. One manifestation of this competitiveness and presumptuousness is his technique of "turning the tables" when confronted with an aggressive aspect of his behavior: he will respond with a variety of "tu quoque" ("you, too") by claiming it is the other who is actually guilty of the behavior, which claim will stop all but the most self-assured confronter in their tracks. Difficult behavior for most parents to handle, it soon leads to giving up on correcting the child-patient, the parents' defeat as teacher and disciplinarian.

What halts the parents is the intriguing question of whether a kernel of validity exists in the patient's defensiveness: i.e., whether the parents conveyed their own untrustworthiness to the child, especially in the area of giving the child his due, reflecting their own unresolved narcissistic conflict. Enlarged for better inspection, we see the child challenging the parent in the common complaint: "How can I believe (in) you when you don't believe (in) me; when you're not even here?"

The unceasing struggle, the sense of having missed out on the essence of life experience, the memory of having lost what was once good, and the seeming impossibility of solving the problem by themselves or in collaboration with another...all lead them to a resigned and even relieved anticipation of the end of it. This in turn in my series has resulted in either a coarcted, anhedonic personality, or a reckless counterphobic challenging of danger, rather than overt suicide attempts, and an ever-present sense that death was nigh. And along with that, interestingly as pointed out by Ernest Jones (1912)[9], the idea of an afterlife and rebirth which is concomitant with the reversal of generations.

III

These preliminary observations already suggest helpful treatment tactics: the introduction of structure, regular presence and control of the treatment situation by strict rules of attendance (in spite of his "more important" outside activities) and a fee large enough to overcome his ever-ready contempt [10]. Lying down also helps to define who's who. The reciprocal tasks of free association and interpretation will have to be spelled out, and the analyst can be assured of great difficulty in carrying them out.

The parallel play nature of their relationships can mislead the unwary analyst/therapist into believing the patient is in treatment merely because he is conducting it, when often nothing could be further from the truth. As is typical of narcissistic characters in general, they will "play" for years without any work getting done if it is allowed.

Confrontations are unavoidable, helpful, and the meat of the early treatment, but best handled by interpretation of aggressive components of behavior and ideation rather than arrangements between the parties. It is crucially important that the atmosphere is not continually one of unilateral authority countermanding that of the patient, but rather a spirit and practice of collaboration in learning.

This means not to let the usual working relationship degenerate into a power struggle between the two of you, "therapy" constituting yourself representing "reality" and confronting your patient with it. This is a sure path to responding to the patient's manipulations, thus acting-out with him the child-parent struggle, and becoming perceived paranoidly as a persecutor, not a therapist. Rather, let the collisions and steam fall on actual external reality, while you as alter ego consider the sources and consequences of the inevitable impacts. None of this means, however, that unilateral limit-setting is not on occasion absolutely essential to the furtherance of the working relationship and the protection of yourself.

The true locus of stolen and discarded part-objects can be identified so that they can be returned to their rightful owners. Libidinal derivatives can safely be left uninterpreted to develop on their own, exactly as one would do with evidence of identificatory processes in a more developed transference neurotic, until they are the source of massive resistance which threatens the treatment (vide infra). One recurrent task is to bring to their attention the existence of two rather than one in the relationships they are (defending against) experiencing.

The (pre-) transference ranges from pretending a genuine object-relationship, to oblivious inconsideration of you as another human being (lack of abiding object-representations), to downright unashamed and untempered hostility (to your frustration of his infantile wishes, such as your appearance when summoned and disappearance when not wanted), to seductive or shaming efforts to manipulate you. There are libidinal derivatives present, but they are usually strenuously withheld from you and revealed to others; the situation with them is analogous to boxers who, only when they tire of fighting, clinch.

Here is one of the central technical points in this essay: mistaking the patient's productions as genuine free-associative secondary process communications to you and interpreting them in the conventional transference framework, instead of primary process actions on you to control and manipulate you, to "work" you, results in the reinforcement of externalizing or blaming operations and relief of the patient's responsibility ala Glover (1931)[11], resulting in not only no change but hardening of his defenses. He is essentially presenting you with a scenario of how he imagines his past relations have shaped his behavior, a self-analysis, which he wants validated by you.

One clue to the correctness of your interpretive work will be the gradual emergence over time of a more realistic portrait of the patient's parents, and realization of what a handful he was as a child; much later yet some sympathy will develop toward the patient himself as essentially a child abandoned within a family. One is really not trying to pursue psychoanalysis at least

"The Bootstrappers": A Contemporary Characterology

initially, it should be clear already. The patient and the pathology and the technique are not really suitable for it.

Treatment consists rather of an intensive therapeutic experience with the analyst making himself very present, palpable, active, and unyielding, and although having a genuine interest in the patient and willing to work with him, by no means able to do so without the patient's essential collaboration. It is a technique of enforced contact, confrontation, containment, and collaboration, not so very different from working with adolescent delinquents (which many of these patients were, or almost were). It is a therapy of aggression, not libido[12].

The goal has to be modified, from a restitutio ad integrum to an improved quality of life, as would be appropriate to a patient so analogously physically disabled. Analysts whose training experience did not include working "hands on" with disturbed children in a residential treatment center, living with them, will be noticeably handicapped. Those whose personal discomfort requires interpersonal aloofness should not even attempt such a treatment, for they will effect only an intellectualized unchanged narcissist. And those whose working view is unidimensionally of libido only, unable to recognize human un-lovingness or aggression are of little use here, either. Psychoactive drugs can play a legitimate part in the total armamentarium for management of disabling symptoms of depression and obsession (for which fluoxetine is especially useful), hyperactivity and panic (imipramine), and mania (lithium).

There is a large element of re-education and re-socialization called for in the treatment, some of which can be carried out with others, outside. On the model of child and adolescent therapy, again, the introduction of a pinch of pleasurable play into the therapy can leaven and enhance the otherwise unremitting work. There is a productive place, I believe, for the escorting of the patient into society and interacting with him there in a relaxed activity such as lunch, shopping, excursion, etc., allowing a different view of the analyst and a less painful confrontation of normal social intercourse to take place. In addition, seeing the patient from a different perspective than his tonsure can be truly eye-opening to the analyst, and bring home how seriously disabled his patient is, though perhaps passing for being merely eccentric.

The theoretical justification for this "real relationship" (Ralph Greenson) or "relationship therapy" (Maurice Levine) with immature patients is the state of their object-relations development, which is still predominately external and actual rather than internal and representational. To put it in (pre-) transference terms, the patient is already handicapped in his development by the physical and psychic absence of his parents; replicating this by the analyst hiding behind the couch is of no help and actually traumatic.

One of the functions of the patient's provocative behavior is to get the analyst to respond to him, to make himself felt, so that the analyst's real-object qualities can be palpated and exert their containing (and later modeling) function. The dosage of this experience is important, however, for overexposure invariably leads to a resurgence of the patient's contempt toward your human imperfections, attempts to manipulate you by means of them, and his own omnipotent un-neediness.

The analogy of nursery school compels itself to mind, a nursery school for feral adults who never achieved the goal of learning to play with other children. The task could be thought of as healthy ego-building through interpretation and socialization, at first the society of two, later more (which could include other such patients).

IV

A special warning is in order: although these patients show a surprising perseverance in treatment, they are prone to abruptly terminate after thinking about it privately for weeks or months, not giving an opportunity to analyze the particular resistance at work. In the older literature, this was referred to as "the narcissist's readiness to relinquish his objects". It can be any or all of: (1) a variety of negative therapeutic reaction in which the seemingly-working patient suddenly and abruptly sours on the value of the treatment to him, out of an envious need to spoil what

"The Bootstrappers": A Contemporary Characterology

has been given him; (2) a repetition of the abrupt loss of the father which is almost predictable initially in some cases, or (3) a repetition of leaving school.

(4) A product of the patient's intolerance of a continuous relationship without breaks caused by both the exhausting effort of controlling you from getting to him, and a defense against (5) his expectation that you will abruptly drop him, as he was by his parent at some point in the past, both (4&5) constituting his paranoid defense against an object-relationship as well as his identification with his narcissistic parent. Akin to this narcissistic/paranoid withdrawal is (6) his finally feeling cornered, discovered, and no longer in control of his therapist, outmaneuvered and outlasted and thus vulnerable to any fantastically-imagined retribution.

Some return later to give the therapist a second try, and, depending on the history, this reunion can be accompanied by elation and a redoubled effort to work with you. The therapist's keeping in touch by follow-ups may facilitate the return, but since the prognosis that the second attempt at treatment will accomplish what the first did not is not good, optimism about re-treatment is not encouraged (though the "reconciliation" is admittedly difficult to refuse).

A patient returned 30 years later to resume his broken-off treatment with his original analyst, having had a similar history of reunion with his absent father after decades of separation. Following a year of hard work, he panicked at the irruption of libidinal impulses, left again and returned, whereupon accompanied by elated affect, his resistance melted away and he was a typical working analysand for awhile, before his previous defenses reconstituted.

He ascribed his changed attitude to finally feeling in charge of his own life (the ability to break out of the treatment compact), and the happy discovery that his analyst had not abandoned him, both a grandiose denial of his dependency and a reflection of growing ego-strength, as well as an echo of (true transference) his life-long complaint that his mother abruptly dropped him as her favorite when she remarried later in life. This patient ultimately broke off his treatment again, retreating to his comfortable isolation.

This reaction is entirely parallel to what happens in his other social relations, especially with women, where, after a long duration of "involvement" of restricted depth, he opts again for singleness after a particular (provoked) disappointment, breach of trust, or enraging frustration with her. Felt obligation to the friend for her efforts, or a sense of gratitude for what time and effort has been spent with him, is either withheld or entirely lacking, and in the social setting is experienced as a ridiculous expectation of him by needy others. After the break, he rues his loss (not of the object, but his own wasted "involvement") and licks his wounds for years, blaming the other for the failure and adding to his grievance-list of having been cheated.

Each such experience of interpersonal failure reinforces his commitment to going it alone, although he remains eternally hopeful the perfect person will come along. It is as though rather than involving himself in a relationship, he is just loaning himself on a trial basis for the other's involvement (the underlying infantile passive parasitizing) which he is sure will prove fruitless (deduced from his repetitious history: the denial of his own need and envy of what the object has to offer guarantees the need to spoil).

After a 5-year relationship with one completely passive and undemanding younger woman, she finally left when it became convincingly clear that the relationship was going nowhere, but still without complaint or even asking for what she wanted. Only after she left did the man consider to himself that he should have told her that he loved her, which would have been for the first time, and that he didn't want her to leave. But he didn't. That would have been yielding to imperfect human weakness; and also doing something.

In the normal course of events, two people having a relationship over time develop a body of shared experience, memory, and discovery about

"The Bootstrappers": A Contemporary Characterology

each other generating a growing sense of familiarity, a progressive dropping of interpsychic guardedness resulting in trust and intimacy, the building of a shorthand vocabulary, and many other such evidences of the relationship having become reified into a structure. Not so with the narcissist, who continually attacks the development of any bonds of attachment and dependency, and starts each day in the relationship "from square one", formally and tentatively, as though there had been no shared history. They are thus as prepared on day 1001 as they are on day 1 to "split" and never regret it.

To the puzzled "partner", this behavior arouses confusion and a vague sense of guilt at having failed somehow, often with redoubled efforts at pleasing the narcissist. Thus the partner is always "on trial" in the relationship, and the narcissist is always given to and given in to. The provisional relationship with the partner can be conveyed by any number of ploys: that you are second choice to the first who was not available (often used with analysts and spouses), that you are being dealt with only under duress (the family's insistence) and otherwise would not be, that you had disappointed her once or often and were thus already suspect, that you had committed the egregious error of becoming involved with her which only reflects your contemptible neediness[13], that you are being related to only temporarily for she is planning to go away, etc.

In addition, the sense of self of the partner is continually attacked by the "double wipe-out", the simultaneous ignoring of or projecting into the partner of the narcissist's own intentions, plus then blaming the partner for it. If by dint of long experience or unusual perseverance the partner defends himself by standing up to the narcissist, he himself feels and is additionally made to feel that he is now exhibiting undue self-concern. This externalizing and manipulating ploy is familiar to any parent, and the patient is unusually effective in silencing and controlling his objects with it.

The typical emotional posture of the patient is looking to the future, alone and elsewhere, and tells of her "good" experiences with others, denying thereby any problems in her interpersonal relationships and thus silently indicting her partner for any perceived shortcomings. She speaks of

"I", not "we". She behaves as though individual people were interchangeable as objects of her interest, and the choice is thus opportunistic.

In typical fashion, a beautiful woman talked incessantly of her boyfriend in her analytic sessions, interminably of her analyst when in bed with her boyfriend, once calling him from there long-distance!

This kind of emotional straddling keeps her independent and insures her from the danger of emotional need and entrapment with any particular individual. The resulting social spectrum may range from a friendless loner, through one with multiple (exploitable) acquaintances but no friends, to one with a single enduring distant relationship which fails to ripen and deepen, thus betraying the absence of two in a relationship which consists only of a mirroring of the self in the other. Individuals are not missed as such, but their response to her manipulative moves certainly is, needed to confirm her still-potent powers; thus such people tend to be provocative. They capture and possess people rather than have relationships with them, dealing with them or not as is their pleasure, exactly as with inanimate objects.

V

It is at the point in the treatment after successful containment and confrontation has taken place that the dynamic problem for the patient shifts: from the struggle with his external object to the struggle against the now-intruding libidinal and dependent transference proper, which is experienced as "self"-threatening. That is, the massive narcissistic investment in the self threatens to be shifted to the object of the analyst-caretaker, with the expected/feared/wished-for annihilation of the self. Naturally this is fought "tooth and nail", and may be the point of final rupture of the treatment, a negative therapeutic reaction, indeed, in the face of growing libidinal evidence.

The combination of increased oral impulses to the object and the felt need to push away culminates in the "kiss-off", the Mafia-like death-kiss

"The Bootstrappers": A Contemporary Characterology

execution of the treatment, which is how he terminates all his relationships. After a protracted but growing feeling by both parties of being exploited (the product of the patient's "going out of his way" for the therapist-object but meanwhile taking all he can get and withholding what he has to give), the tentative object is "written off" as yet another disappointing human in his search for the perfect undemanding and nourishing mother with whom he can be the perpetual infant (his infantile idealization regards with contempt real-world needs and objects as hopelessly imperfect).

This pulling back from the brink of falling in love and need is what terminates his treatment encounters and aborted heterosexual relationships alike, and is a frighteningly novel but repeated experience which was never successfully negotiated in the first place with mother. And I am not sure I have solved how to help him do it with me, yet, either; although to anticipate it is half the battle, as in working through any other therapeutic crisis.

Recognizable anxieties are paranoid/fusion, annihilation/narcissistic, addiction, separation, homosexual, castration, as well as Oedipal, which highlights the technical difficulty of divining which to address at which moment. And possibly it is not even necessary to separate them at the time of developing crisis, but merely to connect the summated anxieties which amount to panic with the predominant defense to all these dangers: the throwing up of all the recent accepted insights and the redoubled attempt to control the treatment situation before it slides irretrievably into the expected disaster.

Possibly in this behavior the patient provides his own prescription: a reminder that it has been too long since a recess from the hard work was had by both parties. To consider this requires a humility on the part of the analyst about the all-importance of his work with the patient vs. his patient's capacity to get along without him for awhile, and a recognition that his patient is used to functioning alone, unused to a partnership.

The recognition by the patient, on the other hand, of the analyst's ability to get along without him (like the parent without the controlling child) is marvelously therapeutic for the patient's sense of all-importance, too, as well as his attempts to control the analyst[14]. When his omnipotence is breached, however, it is replaced by the underlying depression from feelings of rejection, abandonment, and helplessness, which then calls for sensitive handling, such as the special arrangements you might make with a vulnerable child in your absence.

Not only for the patient, however, is it a monumental challenge; the abruption of the treatment can be a devastating experience for an uninitiated analyst, and still traumatic for an experienced one who has expended a major investment in the patient's treatment. If you still harbor the idea of your own invulnerability, these patients will teach you otherwise. To give the problem some perspective and the analyst some consolation, what he is trying to accomplish is having a narcissist fall in love, a daunting task indeed.

Is attempting this challenge a product of excessive therapeutic ambition requiring more personal analysis?...of the necessity to learn to cope with people like this in one's earlier personal life?...from ignorance of the nature of these cases? Or is this the reality of the marketplace in the 90's, the post-WWII years with their lines of people seeking psychoanalysis and waiting lists and patient selection a thing of the past? Are psychoanalysts drawing narcissistic patients of all stripes these days because of their ubiquity in the population and the unending narcissistic gratification offered by the standard technique? As Admiral Ernest King's dictum in 1943 had it, "Do the best you can with what you have".

If the hurdle of the premature termination of the treatment is finally overcome, the analyst faces the challenge of its obverse: the interminable treatment. The same underlying passive wishes which have been warded-off since childhood become manifest in his life in general and treatment in particular, where he demonstrates a kind of "holding pattern", consisting of apparent activity which only endlessly circles without any forward motion.

A striking proportion of these patients have conducted endless remodeling projects on their homes or businesses pari passu with the treatment,

"The Bootstrappers": A Contemporary Characterology

neither ever coming to completion. During this time they are loudly complaining about the inadequacies of their associates whilst living off their energies; the associates complain that the subject never does anything, while they themselves feel "slave-driven" and unappreciated.

The particular counter-transference this controlled inactivity can arouse is boredom and the (acting-"in" of the feared and expected) abandonment of the therapeutic relationship. This perhaps constitutes the most elusive and intractable resistance of all, long after the more obvious ones are worked-through. What is called for is a more rigorous identification of the passive stance and analysis of the particular instinctual aims involved; the problem with this is, of course, that the analyst working himself ceaselessly on his case is highly gratifying to the patient and not readily surrendered even when understood.

This can readily become a re-enactment of the early sexual or physical contact experiences, but more universally reflects simply the wish for attention, which is what we "attending men" (read male mothers) do, after all. These patients as a group seem to have had a history of undue attention in childhood succeeded by its (usually abrupt) loss (usually chronically repeated), the product of their relationship with a highly narcissistic mother. The ultimate (true) transference exposed during the closing phases of the treatment concerns the reaction to (chiefly, disillusionment) and identification with this narcissistic mother, the re-enactment of which thus amounts to the repetition of and wish to recover this lost childhood.

In the case of the male the ending phase of the treatment will prove to be occupied with undoing this identification, thus facilitating the consolidation of the identification with the father, the resistances against which were written about by Greenson (1954)[15]. With the male, then, the ending phase of the treatment is characterized by acceptance of the father (which involves relinquishment of and by the mother, much as takes place in adolescent rites of passage in primitive societies), and in the case of the female, by the taking of a husband, (which involves relinquishment of and by the father, as symbolized in the usual wedding ceremony).

But, paradoxically and seemingly contradictorily, I do not wish to imply that a great deal of interpretive activity is always necessary or the sine qua non of progress in the treatment. For long periods there may be nothing apparent going on, while silently the discipline of the treatment situation is being incorporated into work habits and ego and super-ego organization and structuralization; simultaneously, silent identificatory processes are proceeding in the ego and its ideal because of the availability of the male object, evidence for both of which will surface later on to the gratification of the analyst. As mentioned earlier, these treatments are long!

So, the dual challenge of treatment is his leaving early, or never leaving, and the necessity to strike a growth-inducing balance between gratification and frustration in the therapeutic relationship.

Other countertransference problems abound. The patient's self-importance may collide with the analyst's, or may collude with his usual therapeutic passivity to never become noticeable. The patient's inability to lie down and work may interfere with the analyst's wish for order and sweet reason. The patient's envy may devalue all the analyst's contributions and leave him feeling worthless and undeserving, ready to retire upon the patient's say-so. The analyst's therapeutic ambition may set too high or rapid a goal for a particular patient, or leave him unsatisfied with a partial result.

The analyst's lack of training in treating such cases may leave him resentful at a patient who does not comply with the model technique and requires inventive modification and experiment. The patient at times, heaven forfend often, may correctly identify an operation in the analyst or himself, teaching him something. The patient's ubiquitous competitiveness may seduce the unwary or exasperated analyst into engaging in the game of who is bigger or "pulling rank", or may make just that necessary when you are not so inclined. An especially difficult task for a self-effacing analyst is to at least match the patient's fullness with himself when it is called for, usually signaled by countertransference irritation[16].

"The Bootstrappers": A Contemporary Characterology

The patient's unremitting hostility and ingratitude can wear down the most patient and benign of you, causing you to wonder why you're bothering at all (a highly recommended exercise in self-analysis is then in order, which can provide the missing gratification and assist in the analysis of the contemporary object at hand). Contrariwise, the successfully controlling patient can set up the conditions for bribing you with rewards.

Particularly difficult for the analyst/therapist is the dawning discovery that his patient is lying to him, being "the last to know" out of the necessity of suspending judgment and maintaining his therapeutic attitude of belief in his patient. This discovery can engender a gradual loss of interest in helping the patient, following upon the initial shock. It is the very betrayal, no doubt, that the patient claims he experienced early in his relations with his parent... or thought he did; it never becomes quite clear with these patients who did what to whom, i.e., to what extent he is blaming others for his own transgressions. I don't know if this reaction of the therapist can or even should be analyzed or overcome: perhaps it signals those who are beyond the pale of treatment[17].

Although there is some undeniable intrinsic satisfaction in working with these patients, as frustrating as they are, which can help keep you going, too great a cumulative or simultaneous dosage of them poses a very real hazard to your therapeutic attitude to others. By middle-age I do not think the overall prognosis is good for change in those cases where no attempts have been made at therapy or relationships earlier in life, but on the other hand, the experience is almost universally confirmed (only on or after leaving) as your having made the first real contact in the patient's life and having contributed something very valuable to it; they will be memorable to you, also.

Perhaps the compelling of the patient coming to grips with you and having to deal with you is the most growth-inducing experience you can offer, and, as is the case with the nursery school situation, only time will tell what the future will bring in the way of further development. Some cases, indeed, convert into conventional analytic patients with the accomplishment of enough work and the passage of enough time (which is not to say they necessarily lose their narcissistic stamp; they just become, in the prescient words of any clear-eyed first year analytic candidate surveying some of his prospective faculty, an "analyzed schmuck").

Their awareness of your value can exist relatively untouched right alongside the contempt, denial, and ingratitude described earlier, illustrating the split between the fixated adolescent rebellious ego and the adult relatively reasonable observing ego which is maintained and never integrated. As a therapeutic maneuver, it can be helpful to address the patient's two parts as his grown-up self and his rebellious adolescent self. The dissociation between parallel-functioning parts (one of which may be a suppressed grandiose delusional self) may be severe enough to qualify as multiple personality.

The implications of these splits are that normal Oedipal resolution of the pre-genital phases and their adolescent recapitulation failed to take place, obviously, and that one is dealing with a half-fixated, split ego structure, or circumscribed isolated ego-nucleus if you like, which needs reunion with the rest of the structure for healing. The main medium for this process is the available male to interact and identify with, I believe. The point of fixation is usually the time of adolescence at which they left home (and its childhood analog), rendering the patient only provisionally organized characterologically, labile emotionally but rock-solidly stable defensively, with prominent secondary narcissism.

VI

As citizens in the society, there are some sociological ramifications here that are worth our pondering. A recent governmental study traces the origins of the womens' movement in the sixties to the wholesale advent of their mothers into the workplace in the war-time forties, viz., impairment of their mothering experience. With the burgeoning of social problems which can be at least theoretically connected with deficient mothering experience, such as drug-dependence, eating disorders, nudity, lawlessness and destructiveness, gender-role diffusion and reversal, childlessness, and child-abuse, it behooves us to think very carefully about conceiving and supporting ever larger programs of surrogate mothering (likewise for political and legal forces undermining both familial and communal authority (fathering)).

As clinicians, it also behooves us to think about the contemporary patient population, and the need for specially-adapted techniques to deal with it. Is the transference neurotic model passe? Are disorders such as this becoming the rule rather than the exception? What will the treatment situation become in the future (speaking now of shifting pathology and not evolving economics)? Is it better to have actual therapeutic nursery schools to attempt to undo the damage, or preventative maintenance at home with mother? What can be expected now of new mothers after several generations of this history? As professionals, what should we advise our constituency, and how actively? Can we content ourselves with attempting to ameliorate only those cases which come to our door? Do our beleaguered and otherwise preoccupied professional societies have a challenging responsibility to influence social action?

There are implications for us as psychoanalytic theoreticians here, too. First I would mention the confirmation of the heavy narcissistic bias in the analytic treatment modality which mitigates against therapeutic change when there is both a patient and an analyst so oriented in addition. Next is the utility of considering the (secondary) narcissistic state as a dynamic developmental phase in the achievement of a separate self and relations with separate others, which can be grown out of in the process of maturation, and at least theoretically is modifiable in treatment. This carries an implication that "normal narcissism" in the adult is a contradiction in terms, though self-love, -value, -interest and -esteem are not. (Which may further imply that the theoretical arguments proposed for the "normalization" of adult narcissism reflect the adherents' wish to preserve rather than relinquish their own.)

Next is the explanatory inadequacy of a unitary theory which considers only the libidinal drive in the phenomenon: "Narcissism is the libidinal stage of taking self as object". Not that anyone espouses this point of view any more; they just operate as if they were. To the contrary, this phase is characterized by aggressive and destructive drives toward the object, who is psychologically parasitized. Freud's original duality of libidinal (object-preservative) and ego (self-preservative) instincts seems most harmonious with this view. His later dual conception of (an object-libidinal and) a (self-directed) death instinct turned outwards might then be reconsidered: object-directed in the first instance and later turned inwards under the influence of libido.

Related is the implication that intra-species aggression in general is a product of this stage of development, a manifestation of immature people and nations, and perhaps not a general feature of "human nature". This formulation would correlate with the proposal that the aggressive drive is the older evolutionary instinct, libido coming later in phylogenetic development, put forward in the author's previously referenced paper on human aggression[18].

This raises in turn the whole question of the conception of so-called symbiosis in human development. The cow's relationship to the ox-pecker and its own intestinal bacterial flora is symbiotic; to its tapeworm and its gestating calf, it is not: that is parasitic. True symbiosis is usually between two adult forms in the biological world which enjoy a long marriage. Parasites, on the other hand, usually start their relationship to the host as ovae or larval forms which mature at the expense of the host, rendering a short marriage: many lower forms die after producing and placing their eggs. The human has to be preserved at least the years necessary to accommodate the infant's prolonged dependency, but not without cost, viz. the Scandinavian "tired mother" syndrome.

If the human infant emerges from an intrauterine parasitic relationship with the mother, to graduate to sucking from and shitting on physically and psychically which is also parasitic, to much later enter the stage of secondary narcissism involving separation of self from object which is also parasitic, how can we conceive of the intervening phase of primary narcissism to be "symbiotic"? Could it be the choice of this term and concept, with its purely libidinal connotation, reflects our own defensive phantasy against recognizing the prominent place object-destructive impulses have in the early "idyllic" primary narcissistic union with mother? The English school has been writing about this for years...could the present schema provide the theoretical basis for integrating their concept?

Freud, too, was late in coming to the full recognition of the separate aggressive drive, reflecting our common resistance to the recognition of human aggression. The idea of parasitism, then, reflects that aggression and would seem to be the more appropriate concept (than symbiosis).

Lastly, perhaps the implication that the father's unique role in the child's psychological maturation is as the container of the child's aggression, compeller of the relinquishment of the primary narcissistic union with mother and the secondary narcissistic absorption with the self, facilitator and enabler of the recognition of separate self and others and the capacity to deal with them. Could we say mothers are needed for the child to exist and grow, and fathers for the child to grow up[19]?

Is the father thus the weaner of the child, detaching him and taking the "Mm-mm" or nipple-sucking out of "mother" to render it "other"? (Is this the notorious free-lunch which doesn't exist anymore since the "golden" age?) Is there a pre-Oedipal struggle for the child by the father against the mother, to which the Oedipal struggle by the child against the father for the mother is a consequence? Should we now call this triangle which precedes the Eternal one the pre-Eternal triangle? Is it a different triangle in fact, or merely the added dimension in time of the four-dimensional Oedipal complex which now has a history and evolution of its own? Does the outcome of this Oedipal struggle, contingent upon the maturity of the parents, determine whether the family will remain intact and the children have every chance for maturation themselves, or whether the defeated father will leave the mother with her children, rendering them immature bootstrappers?

Does the absence of the father before this pre-Oedipal struggle render the child a fixated nursling; does his absence after weaning render the child then an orphan? Does the father give the mother child, and then take it away? (To be sure, a derivative of the struggle over the penis, but a legitimate issue in its own right.) Is this the source of a deep-going antagonism from father to mother, and from mother to father? Do we glimpse here parental aggressive impulses every bit as consequential as those of the infant toward his parents?

Can we speculate on the evolutionary significance in pre-history of this emergence of aggressive impulses in the new human triad? Is it conceivable that following the formation of the human dyad under the influence of libidinal attraction, the reproduction that follows augured in the dissolution of that very triad? Did this provide the conditions for the repetition of this same sequence, resulting in a polygamous arrangement in the "primal horde" of early society, which arrangement insured both the protection of the breeding women and the young while allowing the maximization of genetic strength and diversity of the offspring by the dominant male and his multiplicity of females?

And is it conceivable that the American society is undergoing a de-evolution, regressing toward these more primitive "family" arrangements, with our high divorce-rate and serial marriages, co-habitation, single-parent (fatherless) families, teen-age pregnancies, two working parents, court-supervised child/parent relationships, and child-care institutions? If so, it is tempting to speculate on the roles of various possible factors, such as economic (declining purchasing power of the dollar and lowered standard of living), legal and political (empowerment of women in the workplace and out of the home; institutionalization of alternative "life-styles"); and sociological (inundation with diverse and more primitive family arrangements through immigration and internal migration from rural to urban, and the attacking and softening of consensual social values from the aptly-named counter-culture revolution of the 60's.)

Does this inter-object aggression constitute the first showing of the "Death" instinct in the neonate, which later gets deflected from the parents outwards towards all others during the stage of secondary narcissism, only to be overcome under the influence of the libidinal identification with others in the rapprochement stage to become directed now toward the self? Is this the analog of Christ-like self-sacrifice, and the forerunner in general of all religious guilt, self-abnegation, mature concern for the welfare of others, and altruism? Do we see an echo in mature adult behavior when, "out of love for you, I give myself"? This, finally, is where the Bootstrapper is stuck, terrified at taking this very step which constitutes his cure. This ultimate step would constitute the genuine "love cure", not dispensed by the therapist though certainly exercised by him, but rather through being experienced by the patient.

---

1   Horowitz, William S.,M.D., Toward a Unifying Conception of Narcissism, Read before the Los Angeles Psychoanalytic Society and Institute, November 21, 1964. Unpublished.

2   Helene Deutsch, "Some Forms of Emotional Disturbance and Their Relationship to Schizophrenia", Psychiatric Quarterly II, 301, (1942).

3   Because the analytic therapy situation is nothing if not a learning experience, the treatments tend to be very long and tedious, with the analyst finding himself covering the same ground for years. Be prepared to earn yourself a special education qualification by the time you finally finish, if you do.

4   Feingold, Ben F., "The Feingold cookbook for hyperactive children", New York, Random House, c1979.

5   Since the term "dyslexic" is something of a wastebasket category, I cannot say whether our observation represents the true form or not, but what it consists of is a dynamic unwillingness and therefore inability to conform to the society's symbols and usages of language (exactly parallel to the refusal to eat of the food presented and learn from raw perceptual data, their consensual meaning, or social convention), insisting instead on an idiosyncratic interpretation. To quote Humpty Dumpty, "When I use a

word, it means just what I choose it to mean, neither more nor less!" Their mis-use of language is striking.

6   Reminiscent of conditions with care-taking professionals, and the chief source of marital problems among physicians, in my experience. More specifically, those physicians who were first generation (not from medical families) often give the history of the reversal of generations and the assigned role early in childhood of care-taker of the family or abandoned mother, preparing for and long antedating their eventual "choice" of vocation. Such physicians tend to attract and marry dependent "patients", rather than co-equal "colleagues", leading to the marital conflict described.

Parenthetically, as an outgrowth of my work with narcissistic characters and an understanding of the narcissistic gratification inherent in the analytic situation, I have come to the practice of taking into simultaneous individual treatment both marital partners in most cases where this is possible, having the salutary effect in the cases here described of supporting the defeated wife and her normal expectations of her spouse and gaining thereby a valuable ally, undermining his expectations of special treatment, and in the process supplying the missing parenting, not to mention gaining an advantageous perspective into inter-partner dynamics and manipulations. Contrary to what might be expected by practitioners of unmodified classical technique, this practice has worked very well, has not been the source of significant problems, and as a fringe benefit usually preserves the marriage...which too often is sacrificed with the exclusive unitary focus.

7   When his disguised attacks on others are finally recognized by their targets for what they are, he becomes the object of verbal, physical, and legal attacks himself, whilst stoutly maintaining his innocence and externalizing and blaming his victim, initiating his own defensive countersuits, thus continuously embroiling himself in litigation or even less sophisticated fights.

8   The reader anticipating seeing himself in this typology should be reminded that not all under-parented children by any means present this symptom picture . What accounts for the absence of this syndrome in a particular individual at risk is a more difficult question to address, but my clinical impression is that some children are spared this development by never having experienced the initial overindulgence followed by the rejection, rather having experienced uniform rejection from the beginning (i.e., having had a less narcissistic mother).

"The Bootstrappers": A Contemporary Characterology

These "escapees" often present the picture of chastened and over-conforming children and adults, in contrast to the bootstrapper. Some of these children, perhaps partly in consequence of the absence of pathological bonding to the mother, are successfully able to find the required parenting from much older siblings, the families of neighbors and friends, and school, and much later in life, from doctors and perhaps their spouse.

9   The Phantasy of the Reversal of Generations Read before the Psychiatric Society of Ward's Island, N.Y., later published in "Papers on Psychoanalysis" by Balliere, Tindall and Cox, London.

10   Unlike the usual patient who is circumspect or even disingenuous about his wealth when negotiating fees, these patients typically boast of their incomes and net worth in the initial interviews. This is the initial ploy in seducing your interest and dependence, practiced on all potential relationships, which are "bought" and thus brought under his control. This "frankness" is not a product of nor to be confused with honesty, integrity, and forthrightness, for these patients are consummate liars, raising a problem for their therapy when finally realized (vide infra).

11   The Therapeutic Effect of Inexact Interpretation: A Contribution to the Theory of Suggestion, from "The Technique of Psycho-Analysis", (1955) International Universities Press, New York, pp. 353-366. Previously published in "The International Journal of Psycho-analysis", Vol.12, 1931.

12   Horowitz, William S., M.D. What We Don't Speak About: Human Aggression., Read before the South Bay Psychiatric Society May 24, 1988. Unpublished.

13   Reminiscent of Groucho's quip that he wouldn't have anything to do with a country club which accepted him as a member.

14   One patient reports that the analyst's interrupting his treatment on two occasions in response to his stubborn defiance was the most important therapeutic experience he underwent and accounted for his eventual clinical recovery after an intermittent treatment spanning several decades.

15   Greenson, R.R. The Struggle Against Identification. Journal of the American Psychoanalytic Association, II,2:200-217, 1954.

16   Reminiscent of Milton Wexler's technique of out-omnipotizing the schizophrenic.

17   To the reader struggling with the suggestion that not all children are born "good", conflicting with his conception of a innocent tabula rasa written upon by "bad" experience, let me remind him that in certain avian species the larger first-born regularly

kills his nest-mates, the better to insure survival of his own reproductive capacity and that of his species.

It looks as though aggression is a separate instinctual drive, not merely a reaction to frustration nor a phase-specific behavior in delineating the "self", which as such is subject to its own vicissitudes, one of which may well be quantity.

18   Cf. Freud's Totem and Taboo (1912), The Future of an Illusion (1927), and Civilization and its Discontents (1930) to trace the evolution of his thinking on the independent aggressive drive.

19   I am informed that a contemporary ceremony in birthing centers where the whole family participates in the event is for the father to cut the cord.

THUMBNAIL SKETCH OF THE BORDERLINE PATIENT

William S. Horowitz, M.D.

FLAGS:

* Multiple Hospitalizations (e.g. 13 in one year) reflecting manipulation and abuse of the system by the patient (and parallel abuse of the system by the hospital).

* Multiple Drugs, sequentially or simultaneously, all "no help!" (with one notable exception).

* Multiple Diagnoses (reflecting unconsolidated identity). May resemble any symptom picture at any one time.

* Multiple Therapists, all previous ones discounted as "no help", but appeal to you to take them on.

* Multiple (Thick) Chart.

* Patient attempts to control the clinical situation and interview (from the beginning, on the telephone or walking down the hall to the office). Later in treatment, engage in power struggle with therapist over terms and conditions of treatment, types of medication will tolerate (in general, don't), dictating what they need and often threatening withdrawal and suicide to maintain their control (sometimes in the face of clinical improvement).

Borderlines:

A. Have mood instability and lability, not cyclical mood swings.

B. Do have paranoid feelings, are suspicious, defensive, feel picked on and unfairly treated, and therefore due something, giving rise to "neurotic claim". But usually do not experience structured paranoid delusions, i.e., ideas of reference, thought broadcasting.

C. Most of the separate "Personality Disorders" can be found on occasion as aspects of Borderline: Dependent, Passive-Aggressive, Anti-Social, Narcissistic, Histrionic, Dissociative, Paranoid and Schizoid.

The Borderline patient typically is:

* Unseparated, unindividuated. Still involved with parents, especially daughter with her mother, living with, dependent on, highly ambivalent toward. Mother is "fed up" and wants daughter to take care of herself and own baby, therefore demanding of her. Daughter wants to be treated more indulgently, therefore demanding of mother. Sire of baby may/may not be in picture, but strictly ornamental. No reversal of generations, even as mother becomes older and incapacitated. No development; look same at 40 and 60 as did at 20. Ambivalent toward mother and other females, but absolutely intolerant of male authority.

* Orally fixated: eating, alcohol, drugs, demanding. Typical GP unerringly gives benzodiazopines (Ativan, Xanax, Klonopin, Valium) to these patients and they pacify beautifully, as candy to a baby. Their use is almost universal enough to constitute another pathognomonic sign. These substances render them addicted or "psychologically dependent", thus experiencing dramatic withdrawal when taken away, or merely proposed.

* Manipulative: bribe, seduce, threaten, try to make others responsible. Don't present themselves to you with a problem which needs your help, but present themselves as your problem, with, "What are you going to do about it?". Necessitates a therapeutic stance of reflecting right back to them, e.g., "Yes, you certainly do have a problem; how have you thought of fixing it?" Typically will attempt to "split" the treatment team into allies and enemies, whose roles can reverse instantly; like a child, they will attempt to go around the "disciplining" parent to enlist the support of the "indulgent" one.

Superficial cutting of forearms pathognomonic (except in adolescent hospital population where universal). Claim the cutting "don't feel" or "makes them feel", but what it does is make you feel. Prefer sub-lethal over-doses.

* Stable, but subject to transient psychotic-looking regressions which usually recover rapidly, especially in structured hospital setting which they crave (much as they do with benzo's). This why multiply hospitalized. Came usually from chaotic family backgrounds, not merely dysfunctional, with essentially no parenting. Subject to abuse by narcissistic parent not perceiving them as separate individual and a child (of theirs), and the attendant PTSD.

As youths, need residential structured program, e.g. youth camp, and benefit from it. As adult, respond to 1:1 or group therapy better than drugs. Will attend group therapy for years, as the only structure and stabilizing influence in their lives. But therapeutic ambition must be limited, for they cannot be reparented as an adult (a trap for therapist).

* Unstable concepts of self and others, wildly alternating over- and under-estimation of themselves and value to them of important relationships, qualities of people, and valence of their feelings towards them. (Can't live with them, can't live without them.)

SUMMARY

Borderlines are immature personalities, intermediate between neurotics (with their defined character structure, separation of self and object, and internalization of conflict) and psychotics (with their frank regression to primitive modes of functioning, fracturing, or failure to develop). They are very stable in their longitudinal history (fixated), but very unstable in their day-to-day functioning. They have not achieved a complete separation of themselves from others, and their conflicts are external, between themselves and others, much as children. They manipulate others to feel and do their bidding; they often do not feel themselves. And, they are highly narcissistic. One clinical result of this configuration is the frequency of the threat of suicide as a very effective tool, but the rarity of the existence of true depression with suicide. On occasion do suicide, however, by miscalculation or spite.

A closing reminder: DSM III makes clear the distinction between Axes I & II, on the one hand, and Primary and Secondary Diagnoses. They are not the same. An Axis II diagnosis can be Primary, and in the case of Borderlines, often is the more important diagnosis.

THE CENTRAL NERVOUS SYSTEM AND BEHAVIOR,

Transactions of the first conference February 23-26, 1958, Edited by Mary A.B. Brazier, Ph.D., 450 pages

(Book Review, published Psychoanalytic Quarterly, V 28 N 4 October 1959, 545-547.)

The Josiah Macy, Jr. and National Science Foundations sponsored this distinguished conference in which 30 eminent American representatives of the basic and clinical sciences participated. This volume is a stimulating and heavy verbatim account of the 4-day conclave which traced the development of neurophysiology in Russia and surveyed current American contributions to the phenomenon of conditioned learning.

Abstracting the already highly condensed content presents an insuperable task. The format of the conference, with a minimum of structure and extremely active interchange between excellent and informed minds, is invigorating and enviable. Psychoanalysis could utilize this technique with profit. As a chronicle of neurophysiology, this report is nothing short of exciting. Roughly the first half is devoted to the development of the science in Russia, and reads with a majestic historical sweep. The second half attends to post-Pavlovian developments, focused on central nervous system correlates of conditioned learning, on which prodigious amounts of work are proceeding in numerous laboratories. Here especially one finds tantalizing clues bearing on the problems of instinctual and ego function, such as symbolization, pleasure (and pain), instinctual versus learned, memory traces, separation from object, association, and many others.

Pavlov promulgated a concept of first and second systems of signals (pantomime and verbal language being one expression), the relatedness of which to Freud's primary and secondary process concept is evident. The history of these theories and their possible antecedents should be known.

As a matter of fact, one is struck repeatedly by the comparison Pavlov invites with Freud, even to their appearance in advanced age, and a fascinating comparative character study could be done here.

The assiduous rejection of Freud's name from the assembly is amusing, especially as one detects the return of the after-expelled: transfer, association, interpretation, analysis, and motivation have all become useful terms in neurophysiological parlance. More serious is the almost uniform desperate avoidance of the subjective psychic event, in the name of objectivism and science. This would be quite legitimate, perhaps, were these men solely occupied in elucidating the, say, chemical or electrical happenings in brain functioning. However, as one reads, the conviction grows that this illustrious succession of gifted scientists is as passionately interested in unlocking the secrets of total behavior (indeed, belied in the title) as any psychologist, but bound by a rigid tradition and individual defenses to attempt this without the use of a psychology. They seem fated to struggle and pursue their Muse in a cul-de-sac.

Yakovlev, in a tour de force extending for seven pages, gives a brilliant if recondite conceptual model of vertebrate brain anatomy and function, which makes up in respectability whatever it may lack in virtue. At very least this section, and the whole volume for that matter, will restore any sagging sense of dignity with which the analytic reader may be troubled. Neurology somehow has this capacity, just as a study of the unconscious can make one feel sullied. Be that as it may, if his (and others) ideas are a distillate from essentially independent lines of inquiry, then psycho-analysts and neuro-physiologists do have something to talk together about, and the gap between organic and psychic events in the central nervous system becomes a shade less infinite.

This volume is so rich that is cannot be read without adding to one's depth of perspective, humility, understanding, and sense of identity with the human sciences. Unfortunately, it is strictly rainy Sunday reading, and that day seems to be disappearing from the analyst's calendar.

DISCUSSION BY DR. WILLIAM S. HOROWITZ OF DR. BURNESS E. MOORE'S "SOME VIEWS ABOUT THE TREATMENT OF NARCISSISTIC DISORDERS" LOS ANGELES PSYCHOANALYTIC SOCIETY, OCT. 18, 1973.

Dr. Moore, Ladies and Gentlemen:

It is an honor indeed to be invited to discuss Dr. Moore's excellent, thoughtful, thorough, warm and humane, and pointedly unomniscient paper, and an extra pleasure to find in it so many ideas congenial to my own. This like-mindedness, a pleasurable bonus to "normal" people like all of us here, is of course to the narcissistic personality under discussion an absolutely vital necessity, without which he feels in danger of being annihilated. But, I am already anticipating myself.

Let me hasten to add, so you'll know I like the paper but am not in love with it, that the chief idea I miss in Dr. Moore's presentation is his own coherent, even oversimplified, conceptual model of the pathology he is describing. Perhaps this may be accounted for in part, in addition to the author's unassumingness, by his mentioned paucity of "pure culture" clinical material. I venture to say our clinical problem here in Hollywood is exactly the opposite.

Seriously, if Dr. Moore is telling us all kinds of healthy, neurotic, and maybe sometimes psychotic functioning is found admixed in his cases, I couldn't agree more. These cases are by no means unique to our geography or times but universal, unique only to our analytic scrutiny lately. Ernest Jones over 50 years ago wrote a fascinating phenomenological description of the subject matter entitled "On the God Complex", which I strongly recommend for your pleasure. One of the numerous observations he made was the strange preponderance of people with such a complex who took up the study of human psychology! More on that another time.

Discussion By Dr. William S. Horowitz Of Dr. Burness E. Moore's

Rather than recapitulate the formulations (and subsequent reformulations) I presented here some years ago, I think it would be more appropriate to take up a few of the many specific issues Dr. Moore raises in his paper which I think warrant underscoring or questioning. I hope the points will be clarifying rather than confusing, but they assume a certain amount of independent thought on the subject already by the audience. Anyone who has not spent 5 minutes or 5 years with a narcissistic patient may be excused now.

As indicated above, to be sure I also find narcissistic manifestations to be universally distributed, but severe cases not at all rare. In part this universality may account for some of the resistance to recognizing and studying the phenomena, and in part may account for the temptation to rationalize a "normal" narcissism, which to my mind is a contradiction in terms and open to serious question. That the healthy person has an abiding and loved self-image and is capable of enlightened self-interest is not to be equated with narcissism, and is only a distant, if any, derivative of it. The cathexis of the self in normals is not maintained at the expense of object cathexis, is not chauvinistic, to use a topical term; the stage has been achieved where both self and object are cathected enduringly and non-reciprocally.

But, I am saddened to see how frequently garden-variety selfishness is rationalized as normal self-interest, even among professionals who should know better. To obtain a prophylactic chest film or Pap smear for oneself need not necessarily involve elbowing someone else out of the way, and simultaneously may express a mature concern for one's loved ones and even one's community; to load every container in the house with gasoline in anticipation of rationing is not quite the same thing. One can be firm in one's individual identity as a member of a particular gender, religion, profession, nation, or ideology, and at the same time be quite aware and respectful of the others'. Thus, metapsychologically speaking, the definition of narcissism as cathexis of the self seems to me to be incomplete: true as far as it goes, but omitting the particular quality of the narcissistic cathexis, which is at the expense of the object. Mature self-cathexis is not. Here I agree with Kohut's emphasis on the nature of the narcissistic investment.

Discussion By Dr. William S. Horowitz Of Dr. Burness E. Moore's

I concur wholeheartedly with Dr. Moore's approach of developing principles applicable to the treatment of narcissism in any (or all) patients, for not only would this capacity enable us to treat otherwise untreatable patients, but more important for the analyst occupied with the analysis of neurotics and "normals" (including, of course, candidates), such an understanding would enable us to truly analyze the narcissistic residue, which I think is usually left untouched. A more thorough analysis has got to be a more satisfactory one, and, in the case of candidates, will have even richer dividends in their careers to come.

I would differ with Kohut's postulation of a stage of Primary Narcissism "in which the self-nuclei achieve cohesiveness and the whole self is cathected". By his own definition, as well as our own understanding of the undifferentiated self and object, would it not be more accurate to describe the stage of Primary Narcissism as one in which the combined, or fused, self-object duality or unity is cathected? And from which differentiation proceeds, either normally or pathologically incompletely?

In my own formulation, this attempt at differentiation encompasses the stage of secondary narcissism, in which gross aggression (so notably lacking in Kohut's formulation) is directed at the love object, her internal representation, and the subject's libidinal impulses toward her: a truly "anti-libidinal" state of affairs, to borrow an apt phrase from Mrs. K(lein). Of course, Freud's formulation of ego vs. libidinal instincts prior to his dual instinct theory is relevant here.

Dr. Moore's distinguishing the transference neuroses with well-differentiated self and object from the narcissistic situation is of cardinal importance, it seems to me, and too often overlooked in our analytic approach to patients. I have used the phrase "false transference" to describe material which the narcissist presents and the analyst too often accepts as dealing with present and past relations with objects, interpreted as displaced. In fact, of course, the mechanism is not displacement from previous object relations, for there are none (to exaggerate). The mechanism is projection (and introjection), and the "false transference" material must be understood as conversation about the self (and manipulation of the analyst). When repeated correct interpretations of the projective and manipulatory operations of the patient are made, the "false transference" and acting-out taking place within the analysis become replaced by something approaching a true transference (between differentiated objects).

Dr. Moore quotes Kohut's reversal of the basic threats in the narcissist, labeling the threat of loss of the object as first in importance. Descriptively speaking this certainly seems to be so, but the dependence on the object is not the same as in neurotics and infantile stages; it is not a true dependence, but rather a wish to omnipotently control the object. In fact, when the defenses against depending have been worked through and genuine dependence reached in the narcissist, a fundamental achievement has already taken place and the analysis can proceed along conventional lines. I would say the basic threat to the narcissist is loss of the poorly-cathected self, historically and dynamically from the wipe-out effect of his object's poor object-cathexis of him, developmentally from fears of loss of his tenuous self-cathexis through regressive de-differentiation into the fusion state.

I would differ again with Kohut's description of cohesive self and object representations in the narcissist, with stable transferences. To be sure, the defensive pathological organization is stable, something like concrete, but I believe the self and object cathexes and representations to be extremely tenuous and labile, subject always to reciprocal enhancement and obliteration, and regressive de-differentiation into a fused self-object. Again, Kohut is confusing and contradictory when he speaks of narcissists as being differentiated.

I would concur strongly with Moore's and Kernberg's objection to Kohut's "normalizing" the narcissistic state into a fixation point. There is no question that normal developmental sequences can be found in it, and that children go through something analogous to it, but the adult narcissist can not be doubted to be struggling with a rock-hard stable pathological formation with prominent defensive and, I would add, restitutive aspects to it.

Discussion By Dr. William S. Horowitz Of Dr. Burness E. Moore's

Though I would agree with Kernberg's description of the distinction between normal childhood narcissism and pathological adult narcissism, the more important question would seem to be to explain why. In my conception, the normally narcissistic child is on his way in a developmental sequence to differentiating from his object and preparing for separate object relations. On the other hand, the adult narcissistic patient is engaged in a futile defensive and restitutive effort: defending against progressive separation anxiety and regressive fusion anxiety, and attempting to restitute for defective primary narcissistic experience by utilizing secondary narcissistic mechanisms. He is struggling with a deficiency disease, at bottom.

This idea, in turn, leads into another fundamental area we cannot go into tonight, the role of gratification in analysis. Regarding this, let me only say that there is a great deal of gratification in the normal abstinent analysis without parameters, but the term carries with it such pejorative connotations that we are deterred from systematically studying the kinds of gratification we knowingly and unwittingly give, and from developing a theory of its place in treatment. Relevant to our subject at hand, the narcissist needs and must have both a satisfactory fusion and separate relationship with his analyst for cure. Dr. Moore gives us a beautiful detailed description of this process modeled on the mother-child relationship which reflects his non-commitment to a single point of view, acceptingness, adaptability, loving realism, in sum, humane-ness, which must augur well for his patients.

Many of Kernberg's ideas quoted by the author, including his own formulations plus objections to the formulations of Kohut, I find myself in general agreement with. One of his pithiest: "He believes that Kohut's approach neglects the intimate relationship between narcissistic and object-related conflicts and the crucial nature of conflicts around aggression".

Dr. Moore's description of the pre-object relationship with the analyst and the atypical transference are further points of agreement, and have been referred to already. I also strongly agree with the central therapeutic relevance of the patient incorporating the analyst's perception of him

Discussion By Dr. William S. Horowitz Of Dr. Burness E. Moore's

(supplying the parental deficiency), and the regressive non-therapeutic effect of simply joining the patient in his fused glorious state. "This concern for the other, the object, is the model to be introjected." How beautifully and succinctly Dr. Moore puts it. What he describes as the mirroring function of the analyst, perhaps after Kohut, I would describe less elegantly as the supplying of the primary narcissistic experience which then permits differentiation.

The good analyst, as the good mother, as the analyst in the treatment of any patient for that matter, must repetitively swing from empathy to interpretation, from subjective to objective, from being "with" to being "separate". The narcissistic patient requires both, as does any patient, but perhaps moreso – as with a younger child. I also agree with Dr. Moore's prescription of individualizing the treatment: I would perhaps strengthen the assertion by saying that these patients require of us a greater commitment to their needs, and a lesser commitment to practicing our technique. The aloof, intellectual analyst, threatened by elements of a real object-relationship with his patient, replicates the narcissistic parent, leading to stalemate or iatrogenic aggravation.

I am touching here on what I consider to be the most difficult resistance but potentially most fruitful area for exploration, namely, the narcissism in us analysts and our techniques. Only in proportion to our awareness of the narcissistic gratifications we give to our patients in the usual analytic setting, and the narcissistic demands we make on them, can we, I think, be more effective in dealing with the narcissism in them. "Physician, heal thyself."

Perhaps it is no coincidence that only recently, as psychoanalysis has become more secure and settled about itself, is not so much preoccupied with establishing and guarding its unique identity, (i.e., has consolidated and structuralized its self-cathexis), has it been able to turn its attention back to how it came from where it came from, and interest itself in the phenomenology of narcissism. When the day comes, if it ever does, that we can stop arguing about what is an analyst, what is analysis, when we cease

Discussion By Dr. William S. Horowitz Of Dr. Burness E. Moore's

fearing losing our unique identity and being swallowed up, and cease fearing intercourse with others, when we can just be what we are and let others be, and join the community of others...well, that will be the day! Too often, I fear, we appear as the Amish or Hassidim to others.

Thank you again for affording this opportunity to discuss Dr. Moore's rich and fruitful paper, which, as you can see, stimulates ideas in many different directions. I have tried not to dwell at length so as to give the audience a chance to respond, also, which I hope you will. Who will be the first to ask, "But is this analysis?"?

Thank you

DISCUSSION BY WILLIAM S. HOROWITZ, M.D. OF DR. OTTO F. KERNBERG'S "NORMAL AND PATHOLOGICAL NARCISSISM: STRUCTURAL AND CLINICAL CONSIDERATIONS." AMERICAN PSYCHOANALYTIC ASSOCIATION, BEVERLY HILLS, MAY 2, 1975.

Mr. Chairman, Dr. Kernberg, Ladies and Gentlemen:

Although I accept the arrangement of limiting prepared discussion of this complex presentation to 10 minutes, that obviously unfortunately is impossible and compels me to present my thoughts in the form of assertions rather than developing hopefully persuasive arguments, a position I and listener alike find disinclined to take. Please forgive me, then, the brevity and abruptness of what I have to say.

Dr. Kernberg's major contributions to the study of Narcissism are well-enough known to even an international audience to require no underscoring from me. He is one of a handful of contemporary writers who are independently but in combination erecting, brick by brick, the complex conceptual edifice the foundations of which were laid by Freud and another handful of historical workers on this subject. Of all the contemporary writers, furthermore, I find Dr. Kernberg's ideas most often either congruent or at least congenial to my own. However, that is far from saying they are identical, which is as it should be, I suppose, in this world of separate selves.

I laud Dr. Kernberg's attempt to integrate into a dynamic whole his conceptualizations regarding self and object relations, internal and external, and libidinal and aggressive drive theory. It is an ambitious and, I suppose, inevitable undertaking, and excites us to the possibilities of a coherent understanding of bafflingly complex phenomena – maybe even

Discussion by William S. Horowitz, M.D. of Dr. Otto F. Kernberg's

"knowing it all". I particularly find welcome his pairing of parallel internal and external self-object relations, his emphasis on libidinal and aggressive drive components, and his tracing of the multiple sources and connections of self-cathexis and esteem, internally and externally.

However, even as the elaboration and refinement of this integrative attempt proceeds, I am left uneasy about certain questions. I will consider only three.

As in reading Jacobson's masterful exegesis "Self and Object World", the better it sounds, the more I wonder, "Is it really this way?" The first danger I see in attempting such a comprehensive and detailed integration of contemporary thinking is that of re-ification: the concretization of abstractions which gives us a false sense of security about knowing, which yields a structure out of a function, and which takes incomplete pieces to make a (premature) whole. So, while Dr. Kernberg correctly, I think, stresses the multiple and complex sources of the sense of self and the quality of that sense, at the same time he runs the risk, it seems to me, of idealizing and concretizing, yielding a conceptualization which sometimes sounds more synthetic than synthesized.

The second large problem I have with the presentation is its apparent lack of a dynamic or functional basis, though I am certain Dr. Kernberg has one in his formulation. What is the function of narcissism, why does it arise, what does it accomplish, when if ever can it be dispensed with? Dr. Kernberg does stress the dynamic relations between intrapsychic agencies, beautifully, but I am referring to a different dynamism, a cause-and-effect raison d'etre for narcissism, rather than a description of iits phenomenology. (The clue here lies, I believe, in Freud's early libido theory, the idea of self-preservative instincts.)

Thirdly, it seems to me that Dr. Kernberg's (and many others) assumption and sometimes tortured justification of a "normal" narcissism involves a serious methodological question, if not one of fact. I do believe in

Discussion by William S. Horowitz, M.D. of Dr. Otto F. Kernberg's

legitimizing narcissism as an object of inquiry, both in our theory and in ourselves, and in its universality, and in its phase-appropriate indispensability. What I question is the labeling of mature derivatives of early ego-id operations with its original term, with all its qualitative connotations, after those very qualities have changed. I am speaking, of course, about the dangers of the reductionist or genetic fallacy, which I believe we may fall victim to in conceptualizing a "normal" narcissism.

To be sure, there is a mature and normal self and object cathexis, and a mature and normal self and object esteem (peculiar that this term is missing from our lexicon, isn't it?), but, almost by definition, I would assert that it is not narcissistic, i.e., not selfish, not a cathexis of one at the expense of the other, not a predominantly libidinal investment of the self and a predominantly aggressive investment of the object. This was originally the case, it seems but to me, for the purpose of de-fusing self from object, but when the stage of stable differentiation and representation is achieved, the qualities and proportions of drive investments have changed, as Dr. Kernberg himself so beautifully describes. It is at this point, I would argue, that the term narcissistic becomes inaccurate and misleading.

One of the many reasons I stress this point is a tendency I think I see to rationalize the existence of unanalyzed residuals of infantile narcissism as normal and necessary. While I have no final answer to the question, I strongly suspect we can make further progress in discovering whether there is, in fact, any normal mature narcissism by discarding the term, as paradoxical as that may seem. In sum, I would suggest that Hartmann's definition now needs qualification: narcissism as the infantile libidinal cathexis of the self at the expense of objects.

Dr. Kernberg's illuminating clarification of homosexuality I think is an excellent pedagogical tool, much like the crisp illustrations in Spalteholz' anatomical atlas – as long as they are understood as schematic and not existing in the real world.

Discussion by William S. Horowitz, M.D. of Dr. Otto F. Kernberg's

Regarding Dr. Kernberg's metapsychological formulations about affect and cathexis at the end of his paper, I cannot speak; the summary is too brief and abstruse to permit me to understand. I would point out, however, that the very term metapsychology means beyond psychology, means abstraction, and the excessive pursuit of metapsychological considerations, or theory-building in general, at the expense of living clinical data may be used as a narcissistic defense against an object relationship, whether with a live patient, his representation in our mind, or our reading or listening audience.

One last point: I believe retention of the distinction between primary and secondary narcissism to be of great value, for I think they refer to operations during two distinct phases of development having different functions and phenomenology, the former during fusion, the latter during beginning differentiation. But here I am meeting his assertions with those of my own, which I didn't want to do.

Dr. Kernberg has given us meat for years of fruitful scientific dialogue, and we are indeed indebted to him.

DISCUSSION BY WILLIAM S. HOROWITZ, M.D. OF DR. MAURICE WALSH'S "DEFENSIVE AVOIDANCE OF PRIMARY IDENTITY" WESTERN PSYCHOANALYTIC SOCIETIES, CORONADO, NOVEMBER 6. 1969

Dr. Walsh, Ladies and Gentlemen:

We are again indebted to Dr. Walsh, as we usually find ourselves to be, for bringing to our attention an important subject, a subject which we ought to know more about if we are to practice effectively. However, he reminds us about it in such a carefully thought-out way, and so concisely illustrated, that we may mistake important verities for self-evident platitudes and thereby fail to grasp all the richness of his approach. This short paper by my good friend and colleague, abbreviated because of time requirements and condensed out of the author's mastery of a complex subject, is so smoothly and unobtrusively polished as to glow softly rather than glitter. Let us hope Dr. Walsh offers it in extenso for publication so that we may study it and savor it carefully and repeatedly. We must remember that good things do not come easily, but they last.

There are so many fundamental points made by the author that it would be fatuous to merely recapitulate them. Such items as the topicality of the study of identity, its centrality in personality functioning, its dual genesis in biology and psychology, and the various technical aspects of the treatment... all these and others could be chapters in themselves. I feel impelled instead to start at the end of the paper and pick up two points which, for me, demonstrate the high index of value to be placed on this work.

Dr. Walsh not only asserts but demonstrates that his relationship to this human being, his patient, was deeply moving and meaningful for both of them, giving rise to the emotion of gratitude. This tells us immediately

Discussion by William S. Horowitz, M.D. of Dr. Maurice Walsh's

that two human beings had something real happen between them, which is at once the therapeutic task and therapeutic accomplishment with a patient such as this who is avoiding his real self. Typically, effective contact between real people gives rise to and is signaled by a very special derivative of the warded-off instinctual drive, namely feelings (emotions, affects). And when we experience an emotion, it at once springs from and confirms our identity ... identity in both senses: both our unique "self-ness", and our common humanity with others.

How did this come about? I think Dr. Walsh tells us, and shows us, in his other closing point. He says, in all modesty, that he is not speaking the final word, that there are many ways to look at the phenomena, that the listener is as entitled to his own point of view as the author, and that the author, who has a definite view of his own, is both receptive to the views of others and wishing to share with others (which is why he is here today – and regularly). Can we begin to see here the means by which Dr. Walsh undid the damage of the patient's overpowering mother and helped him to rediscover his own true self, actually allowed him to be, to be himself, without fear of trampling?

Underlying whatever technical skills and experience the author and therapist undoubtedly brought to bear, we can see the maturity and sublimation of id drives which allowed him to lovingly regard his patient, maturity of ego which allowed him to regard him as a separate being, and maturity of super-ego which impelled the author to fight and fight hard for the patient's basic civil right ... to existence. Would it be superfluous, or shocking, to remind ourselves that technical training alone needn't automatically guarantee and confer this maturity?

In addition to the direct internal and external perceptions of the self, there is a third route, the indirect external view, "mirrored in the eyes of others", which seems to make a crucial contribution to the self-image. It is because of the imperfection of our self-observing apparatus, and our never-ceasing object-need, that we remain vulnerable always to others' view of ourselves (all of us, that is, except those who claim

Discussion by William S. Horowitz, M.D. of Dr. Maurice Walsh's

---

the exemption of megalomania). In this way we can understand the mechanism of the overwhelming influence of the narcissistic authoritarian personality, who has within himself or herself the power to withhold or bestow acknowledgement of another self. When that self is weak, dependent, a child, it is virtually helpless to preserve its self, except as Dr. Walsh describes, deeply buried in the unconscious. We gain increased respect for the measure of the task when we realize that it is not always so easy for us even as grown-ups to stand ourselves up to these grandiose personalities.

Dr. Walsh mentions, and rightly so, the necessity of allowing the patient to regress in his treatment, with delicate judgment as to degree and kind. Agreeing with him entirely, I would still emphasize that we are better reminded to let the patient progress. His narcissistic mother kept him infantilized, regressed, and unidentified. He comes to us in a defensive state of regression, expecting us to join in dealing with him that way: frightened of moving forward, not backward.

I stress this point because, of course, any technical principle, correct as it may be, is subject to exaggeration and misuse and we have on the psychiatric scene today a point of view which seems to make a "fetish" out of regression to the "earliest" stages. This view asserts the value of regression to some ultimate hypothecated position: not only to what was, but to what never was, a never-never land of phantasy which totally avoids and defends against the concerns of reality and grown-up sexual life. Small wonder it is popular!

Infantile phantasies of various sorts are not uncommon as screen defenses, as was first belatedly recognized by Freud... and they can be just as effective with a group as an individual. The contents of the phantasies are immaterial to their dynamic function of defending against progressive forces. However, many have in common the version of the infant as a homuncular man, simultaneously nursling and miniature sexual adult, simultaneously whole and in pieces, struggling predominantly with aggressive urges. In this confusing imaginary world Orwell would have found his prophecies

Discussion by William S. Horowitz, M.D. of Dr. Maurice Walsh's

reaching fruition somewhat early, for here backward is forward, psychosis is sanity, love is hate, and sex is feeding.

This kind of a "theory" and this kind of a technical approach to a patient does such injury to his intelligence, consensual experience, and contact needs as to constitute a trauma to his self or sense of identity. As in an encounter with a narcissistic authoritarian parent, the patient has no choice but to regress, lose, or better, hide himself, and assume the mask of a false and childish identity, often including identification with his therapist and his approach.

I hope by this locution to have highlighted Walsh's position by its opposite, so that it may become increasingly easy for us to discriminate between this contemporary British foolsgold and the gems offered us by Freud and others, gems which are still there to be mined by the likes of a Walsh.

DISCUSSION BY WILLIAM S. HOROWITZ, M.D. OF DR. ROBERT DORN'S "PSYCHOANALYSTS & PSYCHOANALYTIC EDUCATION" (PUBLISHED IN "THE PSYCHOANALYTIC FORUM", 1969, V.III)

Dr. Dorn has made here a significant contribution, it seems to me, to the growing literature on the subject of what could be called the professional relations of analysts: to turn the psychoanalytic eye onto the body psychoanalytic, to observe, identify, understand, and hopefully resolve some of its recurrent difficulties by the instrumentality of, of all things, psychoanalysis. Not only is the author's paper stimulating and thought-provoking in its coaptation of diverse ideas, but he sets about his task beneficently, reflecting credit on his therapeutic attitude and promising the possibility of healing processes being set in motion. Obvious are his curiosity and wish to understand, his acceptingness of what he observes without condemnation, and his undeniable confidence in the underlying health-tending processes in his subject.

Anyone who himself has reflected on this subject, (that is, everyone) or has attempted to study and research more formally what he witnesses, undoubtedly has become rather immediately aware of the passionate feelings aroused and the heavy persistent resistance attached to scrutiny of how analysts behave toward each other. Both the strength of the feelings aroused and of the defenses erected against them quietly testify further to the magnitude of the author's accomplishment, for the territory he and an understandably few others trod is truly terra infirma.

For this reason I would discount the potential criticism of incompleteness and lack of systematization: each bit of resistance overcome and acquaintanceship achieved with what lies beyond leads on to the next, setting processes in motion familiar to every therapist. These selfsame

Discussion by William S. Horowitz, M.D. of Dr. Robert Dorn's

mobilizations of resistive and curative processes can also be observed in a psychoanalytic group or organization which has taken itself as a subject for study. Indeed, this paper may be partially a result of such processes in the author's own professional group, and certainly a cause for more in the continuing development there.

A more serious reservation might be held about the appropriateness of this forum (small case) for the therapeutic work that needs to be done. Now my view is explicit, for I look upon this area of study, important and imperative as it is, not so much as objective research as therapy. Even so, however, if the literature on the subject acquaints psychoanalytic groups with the notion of the legitimacy of analyzing their own pathology, which we already know cannot be accomplished by merely reading, then I suppose its presentation here is justified. No analyst need be reminded of the necessity of privacy to accomplish this work. (This psychoanalytic group need not be thought of solely as a local society; it might be a smaller group within one, defined by ideological or social preferences, or a larger group including many societies, defined by political or geographic realities.)

Dr. Dorn indicates paths too enticing and too numerous to pursue in this brief discussions so I will take as my point of departure one circumscribed point and return via one other.

Perhaps resistances are at work confounding the attempt to solve any problem, no matter how intellectual, abstract, and far-removed from our field, and perhaps resistance analysis might be a fruitful approach to the solution of certain unyielding problems in our world rather than the blind, futile, head-butting attempt to gather ever more date (and grants). However that may be, one wouldn't have to persuade an analyst that if he set out to learn what happens amongst analysts, individually and collectively, he had best be prepared to face resistance. One wouldn't have to persuade him on this point if it were made distant enough from him, of course, but that is the very problem. The study of what goes on interanalystically arouses certain anxieties (ultimately concerning individual existence, I believe) and

Discussion by William S. Horowitz, M.D. of Dr. Robert Dorn's

stimulates certain defensive measures which in the particular context constitute resistance, in exactly the clinical paradigm.

The perceived threats entailed in inspection and introspection can be conceived of as endangering the narcissism of the subject, which in turn can be understood as self-preservative, the guardian of the integrity of the identity of the subject, and the motivating force behind defenses in general and resistance toward the analyzer in particular. Just as it is the narcissism of the patient or growing child which compels him to ward off threatening aspects of the outer world or of the self for the preservation of the self, so it can be analogized that the narcissism of the analytic group constitutes the resistance to the study of its pathology. This narcissism, then, is susceptible to manifold points of view and approaches, including historic, developmental, dynamic, defensive, pathologic, and so forth.

To illustrate just one possibility: in its emergence from its scientific progenitors and on its way to the development of its unique and separate identity, Psychoanalysis perforce went through a stage of narcissism which functioned quite normally to delineate and protect its identity or selfness. This identity, undoubtedly no longer so infirm and vulnerable as it once was, surely now can allow a look at its "inglorious professional backside" and what comes out of it, that dark augury of imperfection and impermanence.

This approach obviously leads further than can be pursued here; suffice to say, if and when the body psychoanalytic can perform regularly the elimination of the detritus of its metabolism with pleasure and profit (rather than attempting to deny its existence whilst filling up with it), then we need have no fear for the future of any particular professional group. Unfortunately, however, how often since the example of Freud do we see a contemporary "authority" repudiating and eliminating a previously-prized product of his labors.

For a second dose of that humble medicine which the author cites Webster as introducing, namely, the idea that perhaps our field does not

Discussion by William S. Horowitz, M.D. of Dr. Robert Dorn's

attract and hold the very best students, may I recommend an easy and rewarding reading of Fulbright's "The Arrogance of Power"... in which he reminds his political colleagues that they do not possess a monopoly on behavioral wisdom and should look to psychology for new insights!! I think we could do worse than return the compliment. Not only is his title apt and pertinent to our subject, not only is his subject a matter of vital concern to every mature member of the world community, not only will the analytic reader find germinal parallels between interpersonal and international relations on every hand (some because already cross-fertilized from our field), but Fulbright has a great deal to teach us about politics, about the power relations of individuals and groups, about the subject of Dorn's study.

And more: with consummate mastery, modesty, and material to contribute, he demonstrates to us an approximation to the political ideal (and the psychological one, too, for that matter, without having gone through analytic training!!) We experience here a whole man with separate identity but with a rich spectrum of alliances with mankind and its groupings, a man well beyond the narrow concerns of self, a man with a compelling grasp of the world, rather, worlds and peoples around him. He stresses the need repeatedly for us (qua nation) to recognize our strength and be magnanimous rather than petty in our relations with others, exhorting us to overcome the irrational and imagined threats to our existence, so that we can begin to cope with the real ones, among which our attitude ranks high.

This national attitude which threatens to undo us, this "arrogance of power", this national conceit which has us continually befouling even our very best intentions toward ourselves and the rest of the world... this may not appear so very different to a viewer than a modern-day Ambrose Bierce's observation about psychoanalysts en masse: "A group of small men stepping on each other to gain stature". Individual nationals, like individual analysts, are decent enough fellows, I suppose. The rub is when they fear losing that individuality in the group.

EMBATTLED PSYCHIATRY

The Soviets used psychiatry to implement their political ends, in two ways: not only the well-publicized detention of dissidents in their own society in psychiatric institutions, but the subversive attempt to destabilize ours with their complicity in the "rights" revolution of the 60's which saw our insane asylums emptied into the streets, and families with psychotic children unable to hospitalize and treat them. The homosexual lobby used us to advance theirs. The business community is currently employing us to advance its corporate interests. The militant feminists have used us to advance their political agenda. The courts get us to argue their points of view and define their concepts. Popular anti-Psychiatry movements have no trouble advancing their causes with a gullible public. What have we here?

Is our field so amorphous and lacking in intrinsic structure that it lends itself to this kind of accommodation? Is it so fragmented and "schooled" and internally estranged that its parts no longer communicate with each other, unable to defend itself? Are psychiatrists so passive and "user-friendly" that they accommodate being used? Is organized psychiatry so politicized itself that it attracts and is attracted to outside political movements? Is it so preoccupied with its own edifice complex that it remains unaware of what is going on? Are the field's practitioners so alienated that they jump at the chance to be called upon, to be included, in these movements? What has happened to the integrity of the science, the profession, its members?

Imagine a surgical professional society allowing itself to advance an outside cause. True, some of our national health institutes have been heavily politicized, favoring or promoting a particular treatment, approach or institution, but usually in the name of promoting the general welfare. They do not lend themselves to imprisoning dissidents, preventing treatment, normalizing perversions, converting professional institutions into business corporations, demonizing men in general and male practitioners and their sexuality in particular thus making victims of all women, making the men laughing-stock by pitting them against each other in "battles of the experts", or making them out as evil untrustworthy practitioners.

The purely mental disciplines have been under suspicion and attack since the beginning of science, not being "objective" and not dealing with "real" phenomena. This has not essentially changed even throughout the revolutionary discoveries of the 20th century. We are still perceived as dealers in the occult, hidden, magic powers, thus maleficent and not to be trusted: shamans. We are experts in the field of spirits, and try to invoke our powers to contact and ameliorate them. We alone have not been admitted to the ranks of the scientific revolution; even our sister fields of psychology and social sciences claim and are accorded more legitimacy than we. Freud himself strove for legitimacy in his quest for a Professorship and his 1895 development of "The Project" (for a Scientific Psychology). Today's analogue is the resurgence of interest in the "hard" neurosciences, the search for chemical neurotransmitters, and the programmatic diagnosis and treatment approach to mental illness.

Medical specialists who explore in the realm of the unconscious are by definition dealing with the unknown in the view of the general and scientific public alike. No matter the state of the art or science, its subject matter is still unknown, unrecognized, and untrusted. Therefore, the psychiatric practitioner is target to all the psychic defenses, the dynamic resistance directed at keeping the unconscious repressed. What is experienced as resistance in the psychotherapeutic situation is experienced as rejection in the society at large. The psychiatrist is thus fated to be non-accepted. Why he would be attracted to and remain in such a field is another question entirely, but we may suspect that at least an historic familiarity may pre-exist his choice; alternatively, that this occupational hazard is a well-kept secret from psychiatric trainees until it is too late.

Since he deals in the unknown and unknowable, his work is admirably suited to be used and exploited by anyone so inclined. The nature of his work is thus the fertile soil upon which all manner of causes and movements can project their particular ideas which can only be refuted with difficulty[20]! The psychiatrist is thus seen to be a ready victim for any social aggression directed against him, which itself has already been provoked as a first psychic defense against the lifter of the unconscious.

These attacks on the integrity of the psychiatrist, coming both from the society at large and his non-psychiatric colleagues, and the patient population with which he works and their families, constitutes a formidable vocational hazard, indeed. It is something like what the sought-after popularity of the dentist has to endure, but immeasurably worse. The dentist collects jokes to mollify his constituency: the psychiatrist experiences psychic pain which then cumulates in a suicide rate higher than any other specialty, thus further aggravating the opprobrium in which the field is held. On the way to that definitive end, there is plenty of room to radicalize (aggressivize) his own philosophies, join the aggressors, attack his fellow practitioners (disintegrate the field), attack his predecessors and mentors and the science itself, and experience disillusionment and "burnout" himself[21].

It is because of the aggression the psychiatrist is subject to, this aggression he and his work stimulates, his natural antipathy against fighting, and the relative lack of development of the theory and knowledge of aggression in his field, that the psychiatrist is so easily victimized by this intra-psychic and social force directed against him. He must learn to be a fighter. A caring therapist, yes; an intrepid advocate to the weak and exploited, yes; an educator against ignorance and prejudice, yes; a lifter of the veils of personal and social cant and deception, yes; but a fighter in all that.

Jeffrey Moussaieff Masson; Masud Khan

1   A prominent drug company and practitioners who have used their drug have had to fight 86 successive and successful court cases alleging the drug caused the mental breakdown and aggressive symptoms which they were prescribed to treat!

2   Two recent examples are the books attacking both his philosophical mentor and Sigmund Freud by Jeffrey M. Masson, and the anti-Semitic diatribe recently leveled at the psychoanalytic institution by Masud Khan. But everyone knows someone who has, probably himself included, experienced disillusionment in the field which once excited him beyond all else.

(HOPEFULLY) HELPFUL HINTS FROM HOROWITZ

High Index of Suspicion you are dealing with a Borderline in this clinical setting when:

Multiple Hospitalizations (e.g. 13 in one year) reflecting manipulation and abuse of the system by the patient (and parallel abuse of the system by the hospital).

Multiple Drugs, sequentially or simultaneously, "all no help!".

Thick Chart.

Multiple Diagnoses (reflecting unconsolidated identity). May resemble any symptom picture at any one time.

A. Have mood instability and lability, not cyclical mood swings.
B. Don't have true accelerated elation or retarded depression (requiring structured super-ego).
C. Do have paranoid feelings, are suspicious, defensive, feel picked on and unfairly treated, and therefore due something, giving rise to "neurotic claim". (but usually do not experience structured paranoid delusions, i.e., ideas of reference, thought broadcasting).
D. Most of the separate "Personality Disorders" can be subsumed under Borderline: Dependent, Passive-Aggressive, Anti-social, Narcissistic, Histrionic, Dissociative, Paranoid.
E. The Compulsive-Obsessive, Phobic (Avoidant), and Schizotypal Personality Disorders represent fixed neurotic character types, not borderlines.

The Borderline patient typically is:

Unseparated, unindividuated. Still involved with parents, especially daughter with her mother, living with, dependent on, highly ambivalent toward.

- A. Mother is "fed up" and wants daughter to take care of herself and own baby, therefore demanding of her.
- B. Daughter wants to be treated more indulgently, therefore demanding of mother.
- C. Sire of baby may/may not be in picture, but strictly ornamental.
- D. No reversal of generations, even as mother becomes older and incapacitated.
- E. No development. Look same at 40 and 60 as did at 20.

Orally fixated: eating, alcohol, drugs, especially benzodiazapenes. Miraculously, typical LMD unerringly gives them to these patients and they pacify beautifully, as candy to a baby. (The use is almost universal enough to constitute another pathognomonic sign.) These substances also render them addicted or "psychologically dependent", experiencing dramatic withdrawal when withdrawn.

Manipulative: bribe, seduce, threaten, try to make others responsible. Superficial cutting of forearms pathognomonic (except in adolescent hospital population where universal). Claim the cutting "don't feel" or "makes them feel", but what it does is make you feel. Prefer sub-lethal O.D.

Stable, but subject to transient psychotic-looking regressions, which usually recover rapidly, especially in structured hospital setting which they crave, much as benzo's. This why multiply hospitalized.

- A. Came usually from chaotic family backgrounds, not merely dysfunctional, with essentially no parenting. Subject to abuse by narcis-

sistic parent not perceiving them as separate individual and a child (of theirs).
B. As youths, need residential structured program, e.g. youth camp, and benefit from it.
C. As adult, respond to 1:1 or group therapy better than drugs. But therapeutic ambition must be limited, for they cannot be reparented as an adult (a trap for therapist). Some become "Bootstrappers" and parent themselves, a parent/child duo.

Unstable concepts of self and others, wildly alternating over- and underestimation of value to them of important relationships, qualities of people, and valence of their feelings towards them. (Can't live with them, can't live without them.)

HOMOSEXUALITY

The first myth is in the name: homo-sexuality. It really isn't about sex, although they are the vehicles or organs used. It is more akin to rape, the expression of aggressive urges to a same gendered individual via the sexual organs.

The aggression is not confined to the physical act by any means, but expressed toward the opposite sex, the society, the parents, and the self, with destructive acts which have very real consequences in the real world. Homosexuals die young, as a group, from the participation in self- and other-directed aggression and destruction, illustrated by but not limited to AIDS.

The second myth is that homosexuality is "normal" and they were "born that way". This has a grain of truth to it, but not in the way usually understood. ALL humans, and animals for that matter, are born with the potentiality of both hetero- and homo-sexuality. And in the process of development, there is a phase between about 5-7 and adolescence which we call latency, and which is characterized by a deep interest in the same sex and an ignoring of the opposite. So, in these two senses only, homosexuality is "normal", only to be typically grown out of in the development of a robust interest in the opposite sex.

Under the influence of a number of factors, situational, traumatic, disappointment, conflicts, physical unattractiveness, the normally heterosexual individual can regress or go backwards to the previous stage of homosexuality. And he can equally go forwards again under the influence of yet other factors, such as resolving conflicts, beneficial experiences, availability of suitable heterosexual individuals, and the overcoming of the seduction which all too regularly introduces the young into this pathological world.

So, the choice of sex object is not fixed for all time, by any means, and is changeable under changing circumstances. Even the history of having had homosexual experiences does not make one a homosexual in itself.

Many latency boys, for instance, and girls, have had these experiences in the course of growing up and choosing life mates for reproduction. Perhaps the only way to identify one's bent is by studying what preferences exist, when faced with opposite choices.

The next myth is that all homosexuals are the same, representing one immutable variety of life. Anyone studying the phenomena will soon learn that there are several "types" of homosexual which are quite different. First of all, men and women manifest homosexuality differently: women's inherent passivity dominates their usual psychological makeup, although there are obvious exceptions in the case of "bulldykes"; men's inherent aggressiveness dominates their usual psychological makeup, although there are exceptions there, too, in the case of inordinately passive men. Men tend to "cruise", women tend to "nest".

Besides these gender differences, one can identify those truly inborn homosexuals who usually have distinctive physical characteristics which render them uninteresting to the opposite sex and who have a life-long identification with the opposite sex. Probably they have been bent this way in utero under the influence of abnormal maternal hormones. There is another class of homosexuals who are more properly described as ambisexual, with a fluid preference for any object available, human or otherwise; these are often found among creative or artistic individuals.

The clamorous advocates would have you believe that they constitute a significant proportion of the population, greater than the 2-4% agreed upon by most scientists, and that they therefore are entitled to societal treatment as an injured minority whose rights must be protected in law. Simultaneously and paradoxically, they want their habits and way of life to be accepted as "normal". The greatest danger of this group to society is predation on the young, with conversion to their perversion.

WHAT WE DON'T SPEAK ABOUT: HUMAN AGGRESSION
WILLIAM S. HOROWITZ, M.D.
ABRIDGED VERSION READ TO THE SOUTH BAY PSYCHIATRIC SOCIETY

MAY 24, 1988

I wish to thank President Theodore Markellos for his kind introduction, for extending the invitation to address you, and for his enthusiastic efforts to recapture the wonderful spirit of good-fellowship which existed in this local organization many years ago and made working in this community a pleasure. All of us here tonight are demonstrating our appreciation and support to him. In the spirit of the after-dinner hour and occasion, I will keep my remarks brief, but hope they may prove useful to you never-the-less.

One cannot help but be aware of the relative paucity of writing on the subject of the aggressive drive compared to that on the libidinal instinct, particularly in the psychoanalytic literature. While pursuing my studies it was obvious that I was experiencing very heavy personal resistance to exploring it, confirming in a very convincing way to me the social taboo against this subject (which undoubtedly did not exist in primitive tribes which openly enjoyed and celebrated their warriors' bloodthirstiness). This taboo is not only against speaking of human aggression, but even thinking about it, for it offends our self-love, our ego-ideal of the way we ought to be. Perhaps you, too, will experience resistance to listening to this topic. Needless to remind you, 100 years ago in Victorian Vienna these identical sentiments would have been expressed regarding the topic of sexuality.

I intend no offense to any members of this audience with the terms and ideas I offer, and apologize in advance for bringing them up to illustrate my thesis. It is the subject matter which is offensive. Why bring it up, you may ask? Because we are under attack, as individuals, as physicians, and as a society, and it is vitally important to our survival that we understand this.

35 years ago Greenson wrote (Ralph R. Greenson, "About the Sound 'Mm...'") on the significance of that sound denoting the libidinal tasting and intaking of the mother and the emotion of contentment. As we explore the linguistic symbols of bodily expressions of aggression, on the other hand, we are impressed with the prevalence and ubiquity of the sibilant "ss-ss" in such words: shit, smell, sneeze, snob, snot, spit, sully, in-sult, etc. Just as the closed lips over the nipple and the humming sound denotes libidinal feelings toward the maternal object, so does the sibilant hiss denote the closing of the interior and the expulsion of its (airy) contents and the warning away of the object. (The association with reptilian species is inescapable and thought-provoking: is aggression an older and more primitive biological phenomenon than libido?)

Here we find linguistic memorialization of the instinctual act of aggression toward its love object and toward the loving feelings themselves. We could say that aggression, on this early oral infantile level, is the eversion of libido, turning it into its equal and opposite drive: anti-libido, hostility or aggression. Historically, of course, the aggression is systematically directed toward the same and formerly (and still) loved object during development, for the purpose of distancing and decathecting the object, separating and emancipating the self.

This form of aggression can be conceived of as a normal and orderly function in the development of the separate self out of its fusion with its libidinal object which came before, and as such it is a totally expectable and adaptive instinctual process. This is referred to in the literature as secondary narcissism; it peaks at about 2 or 2 1/2, the "terrible twos". In further normal development, of course, after separation has been achieved and stable self- and object-representations constructed, further psychic work has to be accomplished to effect a re-socialization and rapprochement with the object world, one central ingredient of which is the identification with the Other.

When the identification is with another similarly-fixated immature narcissistic individual, however, the rapprochement fails to take place, and we have generational or cultural narcissism. Sustained envy and greed, and manipulating others for ones pleasure, can motivate an individual for life, amassing wealth beyond rational need, e.g., thousands of shoes, hundreds of pianos.

An individual is defined as much by who he isn't as who he is, i.e., by his enemies as well as his friends. The development of one's identity is therefore not only a positive identificatory process, but a negative repudiatory one as well. Perhaps, then, enemy-formation is a regular and proper aspect of 1) value selection, 2) identity formation, and 3) integrity. Thus would the aggressive impulse take its place alongside the libidinal as a source of the traits of the character. Character formation itself, the defensive armoring of the personality (with narcissistic energies), hence would be a general product of aggressive forces as well.

The interplay between the libidinal and aggressive drive derivatives can be observed in such everyday functions as psychotherapy, in which there is or should be a regular oscillation between empathy, or taking in the object, and objective thought, or pushing away the object. A countertransference impairment with either of these drive derivatives can render our psychotherapy faulty, and a balance of both is absolutely essential to effective work. Such an oscillation probably takes place in all human relations, but remains unstudied.

There is another form of aggression which arises, unlike the physiological example above. That is in the instance of the mother initiating the distancing from her infant out of phobic and paranoid avoidance of closeness, perhaps or probably experienced at the hands of her own mother (ala Harlow's monkeys raised on wire "mothers" rather than terry-cloth ones). This phenomenon is often generational, cultural, may be genetic for all we know, is seen right at birth if not before (with various manifestations of rejection of the fetus and breast-feeding), and results in paranoid and schizoid, isolated, cold, and rigid children and adults. They have been conditioned not to touch, so they remain out of touch with others and themselves, manifesting un-feeling-ness, lack of intimacy, isolation and unintegration of the psychic parts. (Cf. the author's paper on WASPS.)

It is in this population that the dynamic conditions exist for deflecting attachment and dependence onto impersonal substances, giving rise to the addictions. To repeat, though culturally prevalent, this form of narcissism is pathological, different, we call primary, and not very amenable to therapeutic amelioration, but it can be influenced socially through groups (again, im-personal). But, all is not lost, for there is a place for such an individual (besides AA, that is), and it is called IBM. This is a peculiarly American invention: a corporate family to enable impersonal association.

Walsh wrote (Maurice Walsh, "Arapesh, the Peaceful People") of the opposite phenomenon, illustrating how loving child-rearing results in a paucity of war-like manifestations in one native Indian society.

For the sake of completeness, we should mention that there exists a small subgroup of babies who purportedly fail to respond to their normal mothers and actually turn them away by their unresponsiveness, theorized to be the first manifestation of autism. If it can be verified who started it, this would represent a constitutional defect rather than psychodynamic aggression. Same for Lesch-Nyhan syndrome.

There is another larger category of aggressive manifestations, generated out of higher level emotions arising after separation of self and object has taken place [such as frustrated love, which was the original theory of the origin of aggression]. Competitiveness; crimes of passion, unrequited love and jealousy; single acts of revenge or sustained vendettas – illustrate the blends of pre-genital and more mature aggression-inducing emotions ranging from sublimated de-instinctualized aggression to cold sustained hostility to hot unsustained anger.

Many civilizing forces work toward modulation of the aggressive hostile impulses, chief among them being the power of love (need), education in habit-training, morality and religion, plus the actual growth and increasing skills of the individual in reducing his sense of perceived threat. But, though the raw urges are civilized or sublimated in their expression toward the human environment (e.g. into sports), some of them are merely deflected onto the non-human environment, resulting in inter-specific aggression, accounting for the depredations on our ecosystems, perhaps one of the costs of civilization. Obviously, the issues of war and peace, exploitation and conservation of the environment, and politics in general (the gentle art of acquiring power over your fellow man), are all relevant subjects to our topic and could use input from our scientific insights and understanding.

The individual who is fixated at the pre-social, or narcissistic, or aggressive level of functioning loudly proclaims his "difference" from the other(s), refusing to acknowledge any commonality, and by implication, his superiority. This primeval assertion of difference is the first social insult to the community, usually provoking counter-attacks from it toward the self-isolated individual. Thus is the basis laid for prejudice against the alien. (Cf. the author's paper on Judaism.) We used to work with the alienated, and were called therefore alienists - any puzzle why we are perceived as outsiders and attacked?

Though the aggressive anti-libidinal impulse on occasion directs itself to the actual destruction of a physical being, much more commonly in our society we see the motoric expressions of speech alone aimed at humiliating or offending the dignity of the other. As R. Dangerfield says: "I don't get no respect !". Or, the dignity of the object in the eyes of others may be attacked, viz. his reputation.

Social or transference manifestations of aggression are generally felt as just that, offensive, but often parentally indulged and overlooked. E.g., habitual sneezing, nose-running, coughing, wet/spitting speech; loudness greater than the distance requires; attitudes of smugness, superiority, over-bearingness and contempt; excretory words as symbols of the substance, hot-air, sibilance, puffery, or actual flatus; yawning or endless boring talk; ignoring you as though not present, cutting you off or dead, speaking over your head or past you rather than to you…all betray the wish for your diminishment or destruction, which is perceived by you as off-fending or pushing away.

Manipulating and controlling, playing or toying with, possessing, seducing, exploiting, torturing, vanquishing, etc., are all common varieties of dealing with the other as less than the self. Typically, after having offended you by any of the techniques above, the narcissist compounds the felony by blaming you for what he is doing, externalizing the process and "doubly" wiping you out. Perhaps the avoidance of human intercourse altogether by the recluse is the extreme example, not so dissimilar from killing rampages against impersonal humanity.

Characterological expressions of aggression can be seen in the typical chronic barking cough, over-loudness of speech (every bar, restaurant, and airplane has someone compelling everyone else to listen to his conversation), and obesity (the latter often drive their cars as if they, too, are enlarged and require others' space), as well as the habits of blowing smoke in others' faces and exuding unpleasant odors.

All this should underscore that the so-called libidinal stage of narcissism, "taking the self as love-object", is, in a conceptual model which is more than one-dimensional, actually a nodal concentration of such aggressive impulses toward the object. Perhaps the clinical point of importance here is that when dealing with a narcissistic patient, exploring historical libidinal transference manifestations may not be as relevant as dealing with current aggressive impulses to the contemporary objects, including you and right now. Missing this point leaves one dealing with the "false" transference and is generally useless, as well as iatrogenically reinforcing of the behavior. Dealing with the aggression not only saves your hide, but establishes genuine contact with the patient, and provides a model of a separate beneficent object relationship. The patient will signal this with "you really have my number!". Delinquent (aggressive) individuals, like nations, come around only when the aggression is confronted.

(Cf. the author's paper on Narcissism.)

Reading the literature (at least up to the point I stopped reading it) one might get the impression that there exist only symbiotic and partnership types of human relations. Anyone outside our field would recognize immediately the absurdity of that proposition. At least in the past 25 years we have officially recognized a state of object-relatedness (or rather, defense against it) called narcissism, the qualities and dynamics of which I will not further recount here. But what is still lacking is a developmental locus and psychodynamic description of the interpersonal relationship of parasitism. This is particularly puzzling in view of the average physician's awareness of the fetal state as a physiologic model of it, the existence of the phenomenon widely in the biological kingdom, the apparent asymmetry of the conceptual leap from symbiosis to separate object relations in our theory, and the obvious existence of parasitic phenomena in everyday social living (recognized by anyone with a live-in brother-in-law, but not by our professional writers; curiously, it does exist in the Russian social lexicon).

The logical place for the state of parasitism can be seen as the intermediate stage in the development of the capacity for separate object relations. It would be located during the narcissistic transition from one to two, during which the psychological need for the supplies of the object, counter posed against the necessity to deny this dependence and the qualities of the object because of the weakness of the self, resulted in the parasitic arrangement: to attach and to take while simultaneously ejecting and injecting his effluvia into the object, taking out the good and leaving the bad in a perfect working model of a tapeworm or a plasmodium. What is being parasitized is the "ego" of the host by the "ego-less" parasite, resulting in what could be characterized as a life-long ego-trip the narcissist is on, living off the "egos" of his victims: inflating his, deflating theirs.

The infantile model of parasitism is that of the nursling suckling and shitting simultaneously. You will recognize an older example of the same, the teenager mooching at school whilst decrying, along with his similarly-situated professors, intelligentsia and the press, the sorry state of his society which supports him. (Again, all is not lost, for it is the teenager's task to attack and weaken the love-bond between him and his family to gain his emancipation.) This also tells us how long the state of parasitism lasts, at least in our indulgent society, and that it is only when consumption gives way to productivity, enabling support of self and others, that we recognize that adulthood has been achieved by the pupa.

The initiation of human aggression toward the mother may be enabled by dentition (Harvey Lewis, "On the Shedding of the First Deciduous Tooth") and collaboratively effected verbally with the introduction of "NO" into the mother-infant dialogue (Rene Spitz), with the natural outcome constituting weaning. We speak of "biting the hand that feeds it". The unweaned have not deflected their urge to feed onto the non-human environment (inter-species aggression), and remain pathetically dependent on so-called narcissistic supplies or emotional food or love from the human environment, e.g. in the case of the entertainer. In this form of parasitism the vehicle is chiefly speech, reflecting its oral roots. However, the addition of the element of primary narcissistic aggression is required to implement the actual feeding on the substance of the human community, which is manifested by chronic parasitism and career criminality. The evolution from consumption to production, then, marks an epochal economic and personal developmental event signifying the culmination of the protracted weaning process in human society.

We wink, perhaps in pain, at the familiar example of the baby or the college student. More serious are the damages inflicted by the so-called "under-privileged", a classic Orwellian double-speak actually denoting over-privileged and indulged, who are supported and given to without obligation of contribution, and who repay us by besmearing and destroying our schools, cities, businesses and industrial competitiveness, national institutions and quality of life, while we stand helplessly by, or feel even guiltier and more indulgent. Ditto for foreign recipients of our "aid". This is where understanding of the concept of parasitism becomes very serious, indeed, I would say vital, to our cultural survival.

What We Don't Speak About: Human Aggression William S. Horowitz, M.D

When one contemplates the enormous support system in our society: jails, the crime bill, drug and food overconsumption, welfare and other subsidies, and the prominence of breast advertising to sell miscellaneous goods, one realizes the magnitude of unmet mothering needs is overwhelming today. What were the mothers doing twenty years ago? They were rebelling in the cultural revolution of the 60's, in large part led by the author of the best-selling book in America after the Holy Bible, Benjamin Spock, who is much more responsible for the protest movement and "me" generation than the official scapegoat, Freud, ever dreamed of being. The so-called feminism movement, more appropriately labeled the masculinism movement, can thus be viewed as the natural consequence of unmothered women rejecting their role as mothers. And with this contemporary rejecting of child-bearing and rearing, the prospect for the coming generations of unmothered children is entirely problematic.

Another group declining growing up and parenting is the so-called homo-"sexual", better termed homo-aggressive, directing their rage at men, women, society and themselves, while claiming their "right" to an "alternate life-style" of immaturity, polymorphous perversity and wanton destructiveness. What will be the next group to claim their "rights": cannibals?

Of interest is this use of "love"-making in the service of aggression. (The opposite is sometimes also true, aggression masking tender feelings, as in pubertal teasing and adult sado-masochism.) In the case of hetero- and homo-sexual rape, the situation is obvious. But, more covert is the discharge of anger over disappointment or hatred to the spouse (parents, teachers and teachings, or institutions) via sexual contact with another, as in, "Eff yu!". Inappropriate sexuality can be a peculiarly effective method of attacking the self, in addition, eliciting social opprobrium if that is felt to be needed.

Perhaps this is the place for a brief ice-breaking digression on sexual acting-out in the consultation room, a subject which highly merits separate, serious scientific treatment rather than phobic avoidance and moral judgments only by ethics committees.

Psychiatrists are fully-trained physicians, experienced in the art of history-taking and physical diagnosis as well as medical management, who are abruptly prohibited from practicing not only the physical laying-on of hands but a significant proportion of their medical expertise as well. To what extent this prohibition frustrates the patient's and physician's usual wish for physical contact, and to what extent it reflects and is experienced unconsciously as a castrating attack on the physician's potency, is a moot point; but could it be that these restraints are part of what is attempted to be overcome in the sexual activity? Of passing interest is the apparent lesser opprobrium attached to such activity, both in ethical codes of conduct and in the formal law, in other branches of medicine, the law, the legislature and government, academia, the clergy, the judiciary, the atelier, the salon, business, and by women. Do we glimpse here a concealed fantasy of the psychiatrist as eunuch high priest?

Could it be that the unnatural isolation of the analytic process, arising out of Freud's and Breuer's counter-transference anxiety and resulting in their avoidance of physical hypnosis and transference gratification of hysterics, actually heightens the transference and human contact wishes of both parties and contributes to the incidence of inappropriate physical contact? Norman Q. Brill, former Chairman of the Department of Psychiatry at UCLA, for the many years of his tenure insisted that his psychiatric residents practice routine physical diagnosis on their psychiatric patients, thereby illustrating that the usual dogmatic policy is at least open to debate.

Another source of sexual entanglement may be a hostile paranoid continuing attack on the trustworthiness of the analyst, which in a suitably vulnerable subject can lead him to attempt to overcome the prejudice with "love", extending himself above and beyond the call of duty to prove his benignity and "clean hands", in the process collaborating in the introjection of the patient's projection and acting-out the feared/expected role.

What We Don't Speak About: Human Aggression William S. Horowitz, M.D

This obviously does not exhaust the broad spectrum of sexual activity, from the purely aggressive seductive patient or analyst at one tail of the bell-shaped curve, through the large middle ground of the universal occupational hazard of the explosive mixture of loneliness, emotional intimacy and opportunity, all the way to the other tail of the curve, the healthily-growing patient and analyst developing real, non-transference, non-aggressive love feelings (which may contain, however, a Galatea fantasy), but we must go on.

NARCISSISM: SUPERIOR BEING

May 7, 1994

Thoughts after yet another encounter with a "superior" person.
(Another portrait of narcissism in action.)

I think of seven such people who immediately come to mind, all with a similar effect on me. First of all, they carry themselves in a somewhat aloof manner, broadcasting their feeling of being special and different from the rest of us. This betokens a certain fearfulness and difficulty in managing social intercourse, for they have little experience with and curiosity about others and little desire to learn from them. Rather, they enjoy being the center of others' interest and talking about themselves. What is missing is any sense of intimacy or personal-ness in their social intercourse: it is purely pro forma and imitates rather than engenders relations with others.

When they talk about themselves, it is in a polished and seamless manner, as though relating a rehearsed script or auto-bio, finished and without blemishes even from an early age. Aspirations, which necessarily reflect a lower status aiming toward a higher one, are eschewed, as are confessions of error or failure. They speak as if they had already arrived at some enhanced status from the beginning. Accordingly, the content of what they have to say about their present or past activities involves their many successes and accomplishments, told as an effortless, natural effect of their unusual abilities.

Sometimes this "glory" is either shared with or borrowed from their close associates, relatives, or institutions. They do tend to associate themselves and identify with larger entities, such as institutions, governments, and religions. A strong religious affiliation has been typical, in which they bask in their self-approved "goodness". This yields an undeniable air of self-satisfaction or smugness. The content of their knowledge is either encyclopedic or focused, but always definitive. They tend to talk in sepulchral tones, rendering their opinions as judgments (casting pearls before the swine?).

Their underlying sense of insecurity is thus betrayed by this affiliation with a larger entity and their fear of going one-on-one with other humans. Their manner is self-righteous, self-satisfied, self-aggrandized, and other-deprecating, thus arrogant. But that very off-putting is keenly perceived by the other as inhibiting contact, degrading one's worth, and unrewarding to continue. It is almost as though the subject's task is to dispense with this new human experience as efficiently as possible, wiping one's hands of it.

Two of these people in my acquaintance have been engineers, more comfortable with material substances and abstract ideas than humans. One of them was an ex-engineer who became a member of the following group, as did another who started his career as a mathematician, yet another as a physicist. The remaining two of them have been at least nominally involved in humanistic professions, but not too successfully, finding their niche in associated activities which, interestingly, involved a high investment in ritualistic activity. All but one were Jewish, the exception Catholic (i.e., you don't have to be Jewish, but it helps). This observation could easily be discounted as a sampling error, but I tend to think it significant, for it jibes with the Jew's historical, characterological, and social mission [22].

All of the people were unusually intelligent; one, the only woman, unusually beautiful. These truly natural endowments seemed to superordinate their self-image and set the stage for the character development which followed: they thus went through life with a feeling of natural superiority, difference, non-consensual-ness with others, diffidence, ease, and self-sufficiency as far as people-needs were concerned. Their fragile egos, as noted, required an affiliation with a larger entity to complete their sense of wholeness or to neutralize the stunning isolation in which they existed.

In only one case was this not evident superficially, but betrayed itself in compelled relationships with other similarly-invested individuals.

The underlying anxiety which is easily inferred is controlled by obsessive-compulsive defenses, which lend themselves as ego-syntonic to the high-level important work in which these people engage. This lends a trait of rigidity to their character and modus operandi, an additional impediment to interpersonal adaptation. Their rigid adherence to their own "superior" values (self-righteousness), lack of empathy for others, lack of contact with the "real" world, and felt non-necessity for learning or adaptation gives the impression that they are ideal incorruptible conservators of values, and this impression, combined with their need to establish an institutional affiliation, often puts them in a position of actual rule, policy, or value-making, having power over the remainder of the populace not so endowed. And, in fact, they gravitate to this mission and enjoy their position of moral leadership and judging (sub-rabbis), for it confirms their superiority and buttresses their distance from their fellows, all the while lending an imprimatur of "correctness" to their operations.

We thus arrive at the picture of the social powers (academics, legals, pundits, government or religious authorities), many of whom, quite out of touch and non-identified with their subjects, never-the-less assume positions as arbiters in our society, whilst being perceived as foolish by that society... foolish in part for taking themselves too seriously. (Humor is not a regular part of their personality, certainly not the self-deprecating variety.) Perhaps this is the implicit social understanding which became embodied in the jury system, wherein the accused is to be evaluated by a panel of his "peers" and not his "betters".

In this conception, a sharp distinction must be drawn between those members of our society who, through their outstanding abilities and efforts, have achieved an earned status, and those members who start out life as the anointed and seek confirmation for their self-appointment. The former are eminently worth having a relationship with and learning from, and they stand ready to relate and share; the latter only seek to enhance themselves by diminishing others. The former cringe at the idea of being asked to judge their fellow-man, but if compelled, tend to be forgiving; the latter relish the assignment, and the "justified" fault-finding.

---

1   See my paper "Let My People Go", an examination of the Jew's role as social and self-critic.

NARCISSISM: TOWARD A UNIFYING CONCEPTION OF NARCISSISM

William S. Horowitz, M.D.

Los Angeles Psychoanalytic Society
Meeting, December, 1964

(Dedicated to Ruth and Seymour)

Ladies and Gentlemen:

I am grateful for this opportunity to share these views with you, for I am hopeful that in the mutual stimulation of a discussion we may have the opportunity to exchange and refine conceptualizations with which, I believe, most of us in psychoanalysis have been struggling in the recent era (during the development of ego and object-relations psychology). These ideas, preliminary and incomplete as they are, have been compelled by the task of meeting clinical challenges common to us all, I believe, and the necessity of making some integration with previously well-established frames of reference, which I am still hopeful can be done.

However, rather than indicating at each step the origin of a concept or its interdigitation with another and compiling thereby a survey of the literature, I have chosen the easier course of presenting my thesis in the form of an essay, implying thereby no lack of recognition of the innumerable sources or connections of these ideas, but hoping instead to focus on the building of a workable construct. I take this opportunity to acknowledge my indebtedness to all my teachers, colleagues and patients whose influence and stimulation are indispensable.

PART I

According to Abraham, what we know as relatedness to objects, whole and separate, begins in the second half of the anal phase of psychosexual development. It is my intention to present the thesis that the normal developmental phase immediately preceding this, that is the first half of the anal phase, which in turn developed out of the preceding oral symbiotic period, is the stage of narcissism, representing an abiding structural and functional entity which can be described, investigated, conceptualized, and modified psychotherapeutically.[1] In addition to expanding our conceptualization of the epigenesis of instinctual, ego, and object-relations development, I believe this concept to be crucial to the theory of treatment of borderline states, the analysis of character in general, and the understanding of certain problems in the analysis of neurotics.

The more one focuses on the problem of narcissism, in fact, the more enigmatic and profound do the issues become, so much so that it assumes the character of a nodal point from which a multitude of other connections can be drawn. These are so rich and enticing that it becomes difficult to circumscribe the topic, a practical problem in attempting this essay. The other major barrier, obviously, has to do with our own resistances to exploring this area "so dear to our hearts".

If the heliocentric theory, the evolution of species theory, and the discovery of the unconscious pose such narcissistic injury, what of the study of narcissism itself? I do not believe the phenomena of this period are inherently any more mysterious than any other, and that their understanding and conceptualization need not lag behind contiguous areas. This presentation will be schematic and oversimplified, as a preliminary communication and conceptual framework, with much elaboration and also modification remaining to be done.

Clinical descriptions of narcissism are not necessary to detail here, ranging all the way from the manifestations in manic-depressive and paranoid psychoses (as distinguished from symbiotic schizophrenic ones) and those found in narcissistic characters, to the epitome of "enlightened self-interest" found in mature people. Instead perhaps it might be useful to seek a paradigm in the normal mental life of the child, and the situation of play with toys and dolls, I think, represents an excellent model. In the developmental task which need present itself at some time, namely, individuation out of a state of total need, helplessness, and co-extension with the mother, doll play (and its antecedent, body-part play) epitomizes, I think, the challenges, goals and resolutions of this era.

In doll play we can observe the childish psychic and physical apparatus at work on its developmental tasks. Without attempting a comprehensive survey of the multitude of meanings in this activity, can we single out a group of characteristics germane to our thesis? Toy play might be defined as the purposeful and organized manipulation of things, usually accompanied by definite phantasies and pleasurable affects, not requiring the immediate presence of mother, and carried out in a state of relative instinctual quiescence.

We can see in it coordinated motor action (control of the body); purposeful and organized activity (ego-directed rather than id-driven); perception of things outside the mother-child entity which can yet be physically drawn into the sphere of influence; recognition, naming, and conceptualization of things; externalization of mental events (ideas, memories, and phantasies) in a concrete and modifiable form; active impingement on the environment (rather than passive reception of stimuli); role reversal in which the child is big and the toy small; all of which can be performed without mother's physical presence, but often in imitation of her.

All of these qualities characterize toy play, from the simplest infantile manipulation of a stick to the most sophisticated dramas enacted by a girl with her doll or a boy with his truck or soldier. I specify these characteristics not because they are unfamiliar to you, but to remind you of the momentous achievement they represent in the psychic and physical evolution of the human animal. And for another purpose: to locate in a concrete way not only the paradigm but what I believe to be the actual manifestations of the stage of narcissism in the child.

In this activity he can exercise physical and mental capacities with some measure of control; he can experience some delineation of his "self" by virtue of his exercising of his capacities, his interaction directly with his environment, and his temporary doing without his mother; he can magically become the big parent who does things to littler ones; he can omnipotently create his own world of things, not just in his head but in the real external world, and make it "work"; he can project and imbue his objects with all the attributes he fancies, and he can have to do with them or discard them as he pleases.

Though presenting a slightly greater challenge, the child in this stage attempts to relate, I believe, exactly the same to the animate objects in his environment, be they his pet or his parent. Unfortunately for him animate objects are not always as plastic, but they can be "worked" too, because they care and they have reactions, and so the little narcissist learns how to provoke.

We have then before us the picture of the victorious toddler, pleased at the exercise of "his very own" autonomy and achievement; manipulating things outside the sphere of his own and his mother's body; giving free rein to his imagination, wishes and power; successfully denying and surmounting his own state of neediness and helplessness, at least temporarily, and projecting it on to his objects; magically becoming anything he wishes, including the parental creator and caretaker; discharging destructive aggression directly or playfully mastering it projectively; and, as a bonus, discovering not only the intrinsic pleasure in this activity but that it is a source of delight to his admiring parents, also.

This is the apogee of that mental state first described by Freud as the "purified pleasure ego" where his world is his "oyster"[2]; behind him (for the moment) the existence of utter need, helplessness and co-extension with his mother; ahead of him and yet to come, the more arduous accomplishment of control of instinct (sphincter control), the intrusion of animate objects with will and needs of their own who must be adapted to, the discovery of the limits to the manipulation of the inanimate environment (harsh reality and the rupture of omnipotence), and the difficult task of experiencing and containing unpleasant needs and affects (epitomized by ambivalence and separation anxiety).

Although the onset of this phase may be more ambiguous, there is some evidence that the crisis for the resolution of this phase occurs, abruptly or gradually, with the achievement of sphincter control, which then ushers in a momentous new organization of psychic functioning and separate object-relatedness in the second half of the anal phase, the locus of abiding identity, character formation, accountability, a work and reality ego, and, I believe, the childhood neurosis. This is an area which warrants intensive direct study, much in the style of current investigations of the earliest phases, for confirmation and elaboration of this construct. From my adult clinical material, however, from various independent sources and distinct dimensions, the age of 2 1/2 has seemed to assume critical importance for the crisis of resolution.[3]

That attitudes and impulses which reach their flower during this narcissistic phase have their origins much earlier there can be no doubt, but to equate the root with the whole mature structure is as fallacious as denying the existence of developed phallic-phase penis-envy because antecedents can be found.[4] These affects, attitudes, impulses and psychic mechanisms which reach their peak of functional identity in the narcissistic phase are, I believe:

1) Feelings of neediness and impotence, giving rise to humiliation (shame, mortification) and envy (of competence and continence), covered by attitudes of smugness, scorn, omnipotence, omniscience, and indifference.[5] Deeper affects being defended against are fusion and paranoid anxieties in the regressive direction, separation anxiety and depression in the progressive direction, products of object-libido.
2) Impulses to exercise power in order to aggrandize the self and humiliate the object, including: to possess, control, command, manipulate, exhibit, reverse roles, spite, foil, tease, excrete on, hurt, sabotage,

spoil, use and abuse, steal, cheat, get without giving, blame others and exculpate the self, invade the boundaries of the object and obliterate it as an entity, etc.
3) The mechanisms of projection and introjection, early identification, denial, splitting and/or lack of fusion, externalization, idealization, reaction-formation, magical thinking, and chiefly, manipulation of reality (acting-out).
4) see footnote[6]

The impetus the child is struggling with during his narcissistic period is to achieve beginning individuation with his limited capacity to do so. The problem is to do so without giving up his all-important needs for fusion with the life-sustaining object. The solution is to achieve difference within sameness, beginning here what will be a life-long repetitious struggle on succeedingly higher levels (exemplified in the adolescent's attempt to cleave from his parents and merge with his peers). The narcissist who has achieved the feeling of "I am I" ("but you are me and I am you") has accomplished an important step, the relevance of which for future healthy functioning cans be seen: it could be called the achievement of individual identity within group identity. Here are provided the dynamic conditions for the first abiding identifications in the ego and its superstructures.

Narcissism, then, in this view concerns itself centrally with the establishment of self, out of the era of fusion and amalgamation of the symbiotic phase and preparatory to entering the world of selves and their mutual relations to come.[7] Much more than an adjectival, one-dimensional description of a libidinal state with self as object, much different than some vaguely-defined end (or beginning) state of inaccessibility, it represents in this view a discrete, organized, normal transitional stage in the development of the self and its capacities and differentiation from others. As such, it is continually liable to regressive de-differentiation, to be swallowed up into symbiosis (more than an oral phantasy, more than a reflection of actual parental possibility, an actual loss of structure and function), and, on the progressive side, preparatory for and preliminary to the achievement and recognition of actual ego capacity (contrasted with illusory power) and separateness – to regulate instinctual need and satisfaction in collaboration with the object and environment.

The sources of the development of an image of self or identity are many and varied and warrant separate treatment. Important contributions seem to come from internal perceptions, from external perceptions of the physical self and its effects on and displacement of the environment, and in a third most crucial avenue, awareness of outside objects perceiving the self as a separate entity. We are, so to speak, what we are mirrored in the eyes of others. It is impossible to attain invulnerability to outside sources of self-confirmation unless it be to relinquish one's grasp on reality altogether.

The self-image, then, in this view is totally dependent on an awareness of the constant flux of instinctual tension and relief through its discharge channels, external awareness of one's own functioning and presence, and thirdly on a constant flow of data from external beings and things testifying to one's presence.[8] A self-image actually independent of "narcissistic supplies" is a megalomanic phantasy (not a psychoanalytic ideal), and the notion can be readily disproven in any sensory deprivation or group persuasion experiment.

But this is precisely what the adult narcissist is suffering from, to make a leap to the clinical subject of this essay. He has experienced continuing interference in his narcissistic supplies, his self-confirmation from others, genetically sometimes from psychotically inattentive mothers, but more frequently from parents who were unable to perceive him and relate to him as a separate individual, a product of their own narcissism. He is engaged in a perpetual search for "self"-stimulation, in both senses, to find the stuff upon which to build an identity (mirror-looking, stimulus hunger, masturbation, etc., are expressions of this drive); the search is doomed to failure for, as with the diabetic's thirst, the supplies never rectify the pathology.

This state of self-less-ness may depend, in addition to parental attitudes, upon qualities in the subject, specifically those that lend themselves to idealization and serve as embodiments of universal phantasies, whether good or evil. Unusual beauty or ugliness can equally serve this purpose, stimulating an almost universal narcissistic response from the human environment: the projection into the narcissistic object of private and public phantasies, the manipulation of him, and the total disregard for him as a human entity...thus the designation "living doll" or puppet.[9] That this phenomenon occurs with certain children not too rarely is no surprise, nor its eventuating in "spoiling" and the failure in the development of an identity and its capacities, one of several courses his development may take.[10]

Conditions conducive to this course of events may be sibling order (first or last), only child, only child of one sex among others, physical handicap, striking resemblance to ancestor, and many other special conditions.[11] The most frequent case in my clinical experience is that of the beautiful, gifted, precocious, adult-like child, especially in the family unequipped to appreciate his special needs and capacities...a not inconsequential social problem resulting in the waste of valuable human resources.[12]

Anne, a pretty 19 year old, came for treatment because of an outbreak of anxiety after having successfully seduced her university professor. Groomed for stardom since a very early age by her mother, grandmother, and a retinue of coaches and tutors, she had up until entering treatment never made a bed, opened a can, struck a match, brushed her own hair, or moved her own bowels, although all these capacities were obviously present and exercised merely upon the therapist's expectation that she could (the latter symptom took slightly longer to "work through").

The role of the ego super-structures (ego-ideal and superego) in the determination of the self-concept and the regulation of behavior is a complex enough subject to also warrant separate treatment. Suffice it to say here, the self-concept, or identity the person has for himself, or the sense of self, or the master self-image, seems to be sustained by a continuing flux of information from the outside, remaining vulnerable and plastic to new influence always (ego-ideal, role-assignment and role-acceptance important here). This knowledge is crystallized in the truism that a person behaves as he is treated, and is the leverage through which a teacher, hypnotist, demagogue, or psychotherapist exerts his influence.

The child's master self-image, modeled as it is after his parental view of him, has a reasonable chance of integrated development when that parental view is fairly faithful and corresponds to that of others and the child's own perceptions. In the situation with a narcissistic parent, however, a bifurcated development can take place in the self-image, one part reflecting a fused and confused self-object image in relation to the parent, another reflecting healthy autonomous self-image formation arising from the child's own perceptions and his relations with healthier objects... this part carried on in silence, so to speak (accounting for the frequent clinical observation of a patient functioning quite well in general activities of the ego and superficial object-relationships, but "collapsing" dramatically in a situation calling for intimacy). The failure to appreciate this phenomenon leads to a very fundamental error in the treatment of such a patient, I believe: an underestimation of the patient's capacities and an acting-out with the patient of his regressive relationship with his narcissistic parent.

This is the situation, I believe, presenting itself to us in the majority of clinical situations which lie in that vast borderline between neurosis and psychosis, what I would call the narcissistic character disorder, which have in one way or another failed to negotiate the narcissistic phase[13] and develop the full capacity for separate object-relations and transference neurosis.[14] In my view this is the common denominator which links a vast group of disparate clinical entities including, among others, the ego-deformations, identity disorders, infantile characters, "as-if" characters, impulse disorders, delinquencies, psychopathies, acting-out characters, pregenital characters of schizoid, paranoid and depressive types (character disorders in general)[15], the perversions of homosexuality and sado-masochism, voyeurism and exhibitionism, and hypochondriasis.[16]

PART II

I would like to focus now on the phenomenology of narcissism in the therapeutic setting. (Ernest Jones' "God Complex" is a beautiful classical essay on the subject of clinical narcissism.) It is unnecessary to expand on the grosser manifestations, with which I am sure you are all very familiar, such as:

1) The patient's bearing of himself with diffidence, mystery, arrogance, hauteur, charm, show-off quality, etc.
2) His references to himself as special or unique and his attempts to arrange special handling for himself, or to perceive routine measures as being especially arranged for him.
3) His minimal amount of attention to other people so that he remains blithely unaware of you and your other patients, the needs of his spouse and his children, or, when ignoring is no longer possible, it gives way to unmitigated furious jealousy and temper tantrums.
4) His unrelenting attempts to dictate what he needs, how it is to be administered, to reverse the roles of doctor and patient, to control the treatment.
5) His presumptuousness and undue familiarity, trespassing and invading your ego boundaries in manifold ways.

With all of this I am sure you are very familiar (what could be labeled the narcissistic triad: presumption, pretension, and provocation). These are the people who do not come to you as a potentially helpful person with their problems, but present themselves to you as your problem, demanding your care and concern. When they speak, they expect a silent, all-attentive audience with eyes glued and mouth shut and appropriate grunts and gestures indicating that you see it their way completely. Woe be it to the therapist who looks away, answers the phone, asks for something to be repeated, interrupts, requests them to close the door, or says, "Yes, you do have a problem". (But this is already anticipating the problem of reactions to these patients.)

Instead, it might be helpful to detail the manifestations of narcissism in these patients' speech, which is, after all, the main arena of interaction in treatment, the chief vehicle of the narcissism and contributor of the most stubborn resistance, and which provides by far the most important opportunity for effective interpretation of the patient's defenses. In this view, it is the central aspect of the technique of treatment of narcissism: although the possibilities of therapeutic "engagement" may prove to be limited at best, breaching of the speech defense is imperative and cannot either be ignored or safely left until later.

Firstly, the narcissist's speech is strongly exhibitionistic (showing instead of giving). His speech may be meticulous, erudite, repetitious, clever; he may obviously enjoy the formation of the word in his mouth and the effect it produces upon being uttered; he may use over-elaborate adjectives, well-turned phrases, light humor, cuteness, baby-talk, fascinating stories, explanations, theories, productions, generalizations instead of specific information, rewording of the analyst's remarks. He may use a flat, boring monotone in an attempt to compel one's unflagging attention never-the-less. The content may deal predominantly with the visual aspect of how things look.

But, more important than any of these and the easiest for the analyst to become fascinated by and to mis-perceive as bona fide communications is the following: these patients will spend the bulk of their time with you describing how they function in this or that situation as from an observer's standpoint, rather than expressing directly to you their thoughts and feelings. Such a patient will not say, "I feel low this morning. It's such a gray day. I got up this morning and, oh, I don't know". He will instead say, "I always get depressed when the weather is foreboding. In fact, I tend to get depressed over so many situations. I am always such a moody and irritable and down-in-the-mouth person. I've known this about myself for many years and everybody has told me this. What do you think the significance of this is, Doc?". In short, he talks at you, not to you.

What he tells you will be blatantly or subtly instructional in nature, aiming to inform you or teach you about how he operates rather than giving you the material with which you can teach him about himself. This is a manifestation of the urge to control, as well as the grandiose feeling that he knows, (i.e., the wish that he did indeed know and that he was the doctor), often raising the question in the mind of the analyst about what, then, the patient is coming to him for.

The content of this instructional material, especially as it concerns past and current experiences with objects, including the analyst, makes up what could be called the "false transference", (pseudo object-feelings which really concern the self) – unfortunately often passing for the genuine article – which can be broken down into at least four components: pretentious attempts at knowing what is wrong when he doesn't know (which may be never-the-less not all excreta), projections of his own qualities onto others, externalization of the cause of his behavior so as to justify and exculpate himself, and fourthly, provocations of the analyst.

Regarding the latter, his words are not so much efforts to communicate on a verbal level what is going on within him and sharing this with you, as they are vocal acts with the aim of impinging on you and eliciting a reaction from you. It is, in short, not concept-organized speech but instinct-dominated speech, not a secondary-process communication but a primary-process discharge. He not only wants to arouse feelings in you, he not only wants to convince you of his view, he not only wants you to verbalize a sympathetic confirmation and affirmation of himself, but even more basically he will try his damnedest to get you to speak, anything, and he will tell you this.

When you listen when you are supposed to, according to the stage directions of the infant-tyrant patient, he is content and all is well; anxiety is experienced and you are perceived as a separate entity only when you take care not to follow the gentle persuasions of the patient. This is the surface phenomenon; more deeply he aims at compelling you to enact with him a specific phantasy or experience unique to his history (which may be quite contemporary, may involve his parents, and constitutes a repetition of the regressive, undifferentiated, acting-out relationship with his object — not yet transference in the sense of a separate object-relationship, but the crucially important repetition in this type of patient's functioning which must be appreciated and ultimately analyzed).[17]

He has the greatest difficulty in simply directly expressing his emotions, but like a tyrannical king with his subjects, wants everyone around him to feel exactly as he does. (" 'Shit!', cried the king, and forty-thousand loyal subjects sweated and strained, for was not the king's word law?") Therefore, when he is struggling with a particular emotion, his main efforts are directed at eliciting in you the identical affect, which, when successful, reinforces his feeling of union with you, omnipotent control over you, and control over himself. Conversely, the experiencing and expressing of an affect which ruptures his omnipotent pose of not caring ("blasé majeste") is accompanied by the most exquisite self-consciousness and humiliation (the function of affects in cathecting the self-image).

These patients are among the greatest provocateurs, clinically or socially. One can understand this behavior from many points of view, but in a holistic sense their aim seems to be to involve the analyst by manipulating his normal attention, concern, and various affects (love, anger, guilt) in order to remain uninvolved themselves.[18] Although they gloat over their provocative successes, they are terrified at the prospect of retaliation, which they freely diagnose prematurely in the analyst, itself serving as a further provocation.

One cannot help but be reminded of the maneuverings of some of the younger nations on the world political scene. If you are perhaps thinking that these patients arouse self-defending tactics in the analyst much more than therapeutic techniques, I would say that you are right, but that in this instance the two are not mutually exclusive.[19] The analyst's natural reactions, tempered of course, are therapeutic, and his attempt to inhibit or ignore them is usually fruitless.

Once having been the narcissistic object of their parents, these patients in the course of time often have succeeded in reversing roles so that in adulthood they play the dominant role in their family, with the parents, spouse, and children now perceived as narcissistic objects. When seeking treatment, they will approach an analyst who will serve in this capacity, meaning one who seems unduly sympathetic or pliant, one who resembles them or their ideal, one who can serve as a vehicle for particular phantasies, and/or one who can be fooled. (During the initial contact, of course, depending upon the proportion of healthy ego present in the patient and the effectiveness of the analyst's early interventions, particularly his resistance to being manipulated, the analyst assumes more real-object value.)

To these people, the external world is utilized as a staging place for the viewing of projected internal imagoes, needs and wishes; as with a young child, the real world is a phantasy place. It could be said that they live in a dream world, that their waking activity constitutes their dreaming, and in fact their actual dreams are often simple like those of children and require no special work to unravel (or are used for resistance purposes to manipulate the analyst's attention). There is a "not for real" quality about them, this "as if" quality corresponding to their magical, imitative, infantile view that to say they are something or to act like they are something is equivalent to being it.

It is exactly as the young child who dons a helmet and wields a stick and is now a soldier. They rule themselves and others by fiat, much as a young government, passing out edicts about the way things are and creating, de novo, with words, established institutions and demanding they be treated as such. This contributes a game-like quality to their activities, a pretending, playful, non-serious approach to their lives and their treatment (and the absence of work habits and avoidance of "doing things" leading to accomplishment and the assuming of responsibility).

The struggle for self and object-control in these patients would lead us to deduce exactly what is found clinically, rather unelaborated frank preoccupation with toilet functions. They have never been toilet-trained, have never submitted themselves to discipline for love and respect for the strength of another. I have found almost uniformly a serious and protracted history of enuresis and/or encopresis, with bowel, bladder, speech, or affect-expressive difficulties persisting into adulthood. The women in my series have all displayed a most interesting sign which I have come to regard as almost pathognomonic: they cannot really cry, but they "wet" and their nose runs chronically, hour after hour, year after year of treatment (usually without handkerchief); the men have shown instead a deep and pervasive passivity, posing at some point in treatment a formidable obstacle to its continuance.

I will only mention in passing to round out the clinical picture, that drive-derivatives from all levels of instinctual development, oral, anal, phallic, and Oedipal, are very much in evidence, but for technical reasons their analysis, as part impulses, ought to be deferred until later (which see). The Oedipal strivings are quite frank, as is everything else for that matter, partly on the basis of the actual reversal of generations which takes place in the families of these patients and the acting-out of Oedipal themes between them, but this too, at least early, must be understood in terms of its narcissistic meaning. Avoidances of conflict with the superego also plays a major role.

After this brief description, let us summarize the structure and functioning of these patients:

1) From an object-relations point of view, they are on the one hand differentiating themselves from the object and establishing their "self", and on the other hand, defending against a separate object-relationship. Fragments of object-relations which exist are usually with a part rather than a whole object, and the object choice is narcissistic.

2) From an ego viewpoint, they are infantile, primitive, relatively unstructured, and operating on the "pleasure principle". Ego boundaries are poorly defined, frustration tolerance is low, thinking is heavily imbued with primary process, reality testing is defective (but not relinquished), and identity formation and sense of self are grossly impaired. The defenses have already been listed. Super-ego elements are present, but conflicts with it are avoided.

3) From an instinctual point of view, they are fixated in the early anal phase, never having mastered and surmounted this epoch in development which makes the major contribution to ego development and character formation (see Ernest Jones' "Anal-Erotic Traits" and Abraham's "Development of the Libido").[20] Lack of instinctual fusion manifests itself in large amounts of destructive and sadistic energies, and readiness to relinquish their objects. The aggression is overt, what is warded-off (split off)

are the libidinal impulses, in this pre-ambivalent phase; partly the libidinal energies cathect the newly-emergent self, but that portion of the libido which is object-directed is merely withheld from the object at hand and given to another (often in phantasy).

4) From a dynamic point of view, they are defending against an acknowledgement of object-need and object-love, which, because the neediness is so great, the capacity to satisfy independently so limited, and the emergent self-awareness so tenuous, seems to threaten to obliterate the sense of self (subjectively perceived as annihilation).[21] In other language, the narcissist is caught on the horns of a dilemma, experiencing on the regressive side the danger of his self being "taken over" (paranoia), on the progressive side the pain of ruptured omnipotence and object-loss (depression)...manifesting the manic defense.

While the terminology "borderline schizophrenia" is often used, borderline[22] patients actually show important differences from the schizophrenic group. You are familiar with the frequent problem of handling the family of a schizophrenic patient, stemming from the symbiotic relationship between the patient and his parent, and the disturbance ensuing from the introduction of a third party, the therapist. In striking contrast to this, my clinical experience with borderlines has been noteworthy in that I have never been contacted once by a parent or spouse. Indeed, one could observe at times the patient vainly manipulating the analyst and parent to get involved with each other. Parental reactions seem to be along the line of being quite content to be relieved of the responsibility of dealing with the patient.

Another impressive difference is the therapeutic strategy which works in these two kinds of cases. According to Milton Wexler, the therapeutic task with schizophrenics is to facilitate the building up of a good internal object by presenting oneself in as assimilable a form as possible. It seems to me that with borderlines, the strategy which works, when it does[23], is somewhat different: to so present yourself as to make impossible the patient's attempt to evade a relationship with you through narcissistic defenses — to compel him to come to grips with you, to get involved with you, to relate to you. This entails, I think, less emphasis on one's palatability, less passivity and non-commitment, more active confrontation, intervention, limit-setting (more by confrontation with attitudes than prohibition of actions) and interpretation, focusing specifically on the patient's defenses against an object-relationship.

At this point it becomes necessary to at least make note of the narcissistic elements in the treatment situation, an awareness of which is essential to successful engagement of these patients. Besides the contributions of the patient, which in the case of any sick and regressed person is considerable and in the case of narcissistic people is of paramount importance, there are the contributions of both the analyst and the therapeutic setting itself.

That the attempt to change or cure a person, especially a very sick one, has omnipotent implications goes without saying – I'm afraid all too often. That we set time aside for the patient which is only his, that we devote our attention and understanding to him without demanding a return (even making it easier for him to ignore us), that we implicitly promise ourselves for as long as is necessary, these and many other qualities constitute the essence of narcissistic gratification — in which the analyst is the needed but possessed and ignored object.

What for the neurotic patient in the therapeutic situation constitutes abstinence, for the narcissistic patient constitutes gratification. The implications of this in the general theory of technique, in fact the whole issue of narcissism in psychoanalysis, goes far afield of this essay; suffice it to say, these very narcissistic qualities pose by far the greatest impediment to the successful resolution of narcissistic defense in any patient.

Although it is impossible to generalize about such a wide assortment of diagnostic entities, it will be clear, I think, that classical psychoanalysis may not be the treatment of choice for some of these patients initially. Firstly, the presentation of the analyst as a real object and the task of helping the patient to deal with him may or may not be consonant with classical technique and may require major modifications to be accomplished (depending on one's definition). Secondly, classical analysis provides much too much narcissistic gratification for some of these patients, in which they revel and play enthusiastically without, however, any real psychotherapeutic work being accomplished.

Thirdly, while in the case of transference neurotics the roles of patient and analyst are more-or-less taken for granted and they can "relax" and "analyze" pieces of psychic content, in the case of narcissists these conditions are lacking and the identities, roles and functions of the two parties are continually at issue. Coming to grips with the two "selves" involved and their interaction is not only immediately necessary, but has a salutary integrating effect on the patient; examining fragments has a disorganizing effect. (Said another way, the neurotic has an ego which can be therapeutically split to consider internalized conflicts; the narcissist does not yet have this ego and is in a prestage of conflict, externalizing and struggling with his object.)

When the narcissistic defenses have given way to what lies beneath (or ahead)...depression, anxiety, conflict, and an infantile need for the therapist...then the therapeutic situation has made a fundamental change and the classical technique of analysis has some promise of accomplishing something. This "conversion" is the same that takes place in any character neurosis when, after a period of treatment, it becomes transformed into an unfrozen, living neurosis.[24]

The preliminary work can be performed in a variety of ways, depending on the patient and circumstances, ranging all the way from spaced interviews vis-à-vis to daily interview using the couch, i.e., psychotherapy to unmodified analysis, sometimes progressively in this order. On those occasions where I have attempted to reverse this sequence in the face of mounting anxiety by sitting up the patient or reducing frequency, rather than interpreting more pertinently, it has proven to be a mistake, the patient seizing upon this "break" in the analyst's consistency to use it for manipulatory purposes, to assume control of the treatment, and shortly to withdraw (i.e., a tight rein must be kept).[25]

The therapeutic risk, then, is that these patients will try to convert the treatment situation into a narcissistic gratification and have nothing happen therapeutically, or turn away in narcissistic frustration. The therapeutic task, then, is to bring about a genuine object-relationship with you; to facilitate it, to compel it, to block efforts to avoid it (in a resistive rather than intrusive sense). In the introductory interviews, careful attention must be paid to why he is coming (is he suffering?), why to you, what he hopes to gain and what he expects to give, how he visualizes the treatment process and in what way he expects the help to be given. (The roles and issues must be contended with right from the beginning.) Considerations regarding time and money must be especially carefully scrutinized, for in my experience most often these are the carriers of silent phantasies which, when gratified, nullify whatever else may seem to be going on in the treatment.

Perhaps with no other general class of patients do arise so starkly the issues of the patient's and the analyst's privileges and obligations, with of course the patient wanting the lion's share of the former and none of the latter. The analyst must have a firm notion of his own role, and what is involved in patienthood, firm to the point of unassailable conviction; it must reflect in his behavior, and very often it must be made explicit. This calls, of course, for a very firm sense of identity in the analyst and a healthy enough appreciation of his external objects to keep them "in their place" and himself in his. These patients as children often have never been put in their place, and they will verbalize this.

What I am describing might be analogized on the model of a good substitute teacher who, never having met his class before, never-the-less has a firm idea of his own and his pupils' positions, does not succumb passively and ingratiatingly to their intimidating and testing him, nor react with authoritarian strictness, but has the situation in hand and proceeds to attend to the work seriously, but not without humor. (Incidentally, humor is extremely effective with these people and sometimes the more pointed and even sarcastic the interpretation, the better.) The point here is that you present yourself as a firm, discrete, separate object, easily palpable by the patient, your limits are easily defined (and you help him define his), and further, you are a separate object who is interested in him, but neither loves nor hates him (neither wet-nurse nor persecutor, though probably tapping masculine more than feminine identifications in the analyst).

This, then, is the posture of the analyst, and hopefully not an assumed one but integrated into his professional identity. What of his specific verbal activity? During the preparatory phase, this consists predominately of a repeated and consistent demonstration and verbalization of the patient's particular narcissistic wishes, need, expectations, phantasies, convictions (even transient delusions), wherever they make their appearance, but in particular in his relationship to you.[26]

Although identifying the particular impulse is important for affective contact, the emphasis here is on what he wants to do to you (the object). One interesting observation is that these attitudes, long ago relinquished by us, are quite active and relatively un-defended in these patients; their confrontation is not only not denied, but is received with a feeling of great pleasure and usually laughter. Not only does it yield a narcissistic bonus to them that you know about these obvious but socially-unspoken attitudes, but even more important, it is felt as a point of real contact and understanding and attention to them (genuine object-cathexis) and is received with real gratitude [27], (though cumulatively there may be a risk of excessive narcissistic injury with feelings of persecution). It also provides a model to them for later identification of a separate strong object having genuine object-cathexis of another person. They will communicate this recognition by saying, "You are the only person who really know me, who really has my 'number' ".

Later more traditional interpretations of affect, impulse and defense become appropriate as more functioning ego is built and/or uncovered. At first these will concern themselves with oral and anal and super-ego issues, naturally. You will note the omission of reference to interpreting either libidinal impulses or genetic transference material. It appears advisable to forget about these issues for some period of time, even though the patient will present you with all kinds of tempting material susceptible of such "interpretation", and concentrate on aggressive and selfish wishes toward current objects, usually in projected form. When the "conversion" finally takes place, object-libido, anxiety, and a good working relationship will reward the analyst with the ingredients for his traditional techniques.

I have attempted to survey, I'm afraid, too broad a field involving many complicated issues. Obviously, a great deal has been left out and much has been oversimplified, I'm sure at times to the point of injustice. Hopefully, however, perhaps I have communicated to you some feel of how I think about these patients and what I do.

Reactions to these patients are many and varied, as could be expected. Realistic reactions stem from the patient's efforts to provoke, to challenge the integrity of the analyst's identity, and to manipulate his interest. In addition, these patients are unpleasant, ungiving, and monotonously uniform (because not yet individuated), and have the capacity to be actually destructive to you.

They have a special capacity to arouse counter-transference reactions, moreover, precisely because of the narcissistic elements present, based on the analyst's own relations to a very special current and past object: himself. The history of how he resolved his own infantile narcissism, how abruptly it underwent repression, how vigorously reaction formations were erected against it, what particular sublimations he developed for it, will determine in a general way how he deals with the narcissism in others and threats to his own.

Probably, I think, there are three reaction types. Those with strong reaction formations will tend to assume a superego attitude toward the patient, with strictness, condemnation, disgust, rejection, and overactivity. Others will display an id attitude, subtly or quite consciously enjoying and encouraging, not intervening and indulging the narcissism of their patients. Worse yet than either of these is the narcissistic attitude of ignoring the patient and treating him with contempt while simultaneously projecting this narcissism into him, doubly wiping him out. Of course, we are all striving for the rational course: an ego attitude which reflects recognition of reality, adaptation to it, and reconciliation with it.

Thank you.

1	The narcissism I speak of has been referred to in the classical literature as secondary. For orientation, I refer to the mental state of undifferentiation from object as symbiosis (primary narcissism), the state of beginning differentiation from object as narcissism (secondary narcissism), and the state of relatively complete differentiation with autonomy as the stage of object-relatedness.

This is gross and descriptive, to be sure, does not yet take into account the overlapping of stages nor the locus and qualities of internal object representations, but does provide two distinct advantages: it constructs a genetic series in the development of object-relations parallel to and potentially correlatable with stages in psychosexual development, and secondly, it eliminates the conceptual bias (itself narcissistic) of equating internal events (phantasies and strivings) with external actuality, e.g., the child's wishes to function autonomously and his belief that he is, in fact, relating to separate objects precedes his actual capacity to do so.

In this view, primary and secondary narcissism are virtual polar opposites, the former referring to the state of fusion, the latter to the state of beginning differentiation (this alone would seem to qualify the usefulness of these terms). To sum, symbiosis could be defined as the stage in which the self is cathected by virtue of cathexis of the object, narcissism as the stage in which the self is cathected at the expense of the object, and object-relatedness as the stage in which self and object are cathected independently and enduringly.

2	The perigee seems to be uncontrollable instinctual urge, i.e. excretory incontinence.

3	It is at this point, interestingly, when regular bowel function is established that a time sense begins. The narcissist still lives in a timeless world, subjectively in limbo, and it is often reflected in a youthful countenance; "engagement" in the world of reality renders him a "real" person, to himself and his fellows.

4	The contemporary concern with the earliest phases of psychic life, albeit the most inscrutable, seems to me to represent an impulse which can be understood as well as argued: namely, the wish for mystical re-union and re-birth, one of a variety of narcissistic phantasies patient and doctor alike may harbor. Not surprisingly, narcissistic elements abound in psychoanalysis, one obvious residual of which cannot have escaped your attention: the technical term we reserve for the need-fulfilling, sought-after, loving, caretaking, living and breathing whole human being: object.

5   This results in the pathognomonic attitude of the narcissist: "I don't care, who needs it, who needs you?", or more colloquially and accurately, "I don't give a shit!". Saying no to need and object = identity.

6   I have the impression that characteristic of this period is a limited but universal set of phantasies, which bear some cogent relationship with dramaturgy and its set of plots. Drama may represent the artistic sublimation of the narcissistic period.

7   The vicissitudes of the concept of "self" in the history of psychoanalysis would itself make a fascinating chapter. The German "Ich" and Latin-English "Ego" both refer to the "I". Shortly, the ego was depersonalized and mechanized into a set of functions, while simultaneously it was personified in its relations to the other structures. Only recently have these come together in a revival of interest in the ego and the self.

8   Crucial to this thesis is the idea that parallel to the internal process called cathexis of an object-representation is an external process of attention to the actual human being which, proportionate to the intensity and quality, yields a faithful perception of the qualities of the object, and most important, is actually perceived by the object, feeding or stimulating his own self-cathexis. By-passing the vexing question of whether the psychic apparatus is an open or closed energic system, i.e., whether it can receive quanta of energy from the outside, phenomenologically at least, it seems our self-cathexis is susceptible to outside stimulation.

9   I refer here to the almost universal latent capacity which finds typical expression in hero worship, royalty and celebrity awe. Otherwise normal and well-behaved people will either invade the object's privacy in varying degrees, or fail to react at all, sometimes talking in their presence as though they did not exist (a common experience among "show people") – exactly as with a young child.

10   Such a victim may attempt to comply with the introjected phantasies and become the partner in the family's and society's acting-out (professional actors and certain delinquents), may rebel and attempt to "de-idealize" himself to establish his identity (normal in anal phase of childhood and adolescence, certain other kinds of delinquents), or may withdraw from the repeated insults to the integrity of his identity (as for instance in the case of certain misanthropic wealthy people).

11   Whether there are cultural, geographic, ethnic, or professional biases toward the narcissistic treatment of children seems a moot point, though an easily demonstrable factor in the "other fellow's" family.

12   Probably there is an almost universal bias in the direction of treating females as less than complete and separate people, a product of unresolved castration anxiety, which often leads to narcissistic fixation. In "normal" amounts, however, this is not without its eventual social usefulness in bearing and rearing children.

13   This conceptualization of narcissism bears some relationship seemingly to the existential school's state of "estrangement" and the object-relations school's concept of "schizoid position", which begs for fuller elaboration.

14   The concept of transference arose in an historical setting which took for granted what we now identify as the capacity for object-relatedness, Freud himself later distinguishing transference from narcissistic neuroses. It is implicit in the definition which includes temporal displacement of attitudes from past toward the current object: analyst. Though of course the concept can be extended and re-defined in any useful way, to make it synonymous with any of the variety of repetitions the psyche experiences is to rob it of specific meaning. I would distinguish transference as that particular form of repetitive object relationship found in the analytic situation after individuation (from object) has taken place, and the capacities developed for distinguishing past from present, remembering past objects and recognizing current ones. Traditional "transference" interpretations are clinically meaningless without these criteria.

One encounters similar conceptual difficulties regarding transference with adult narcissists as with children in treatment, with whom relations with the parents are a current reality (similar also in reluctance to freely associate, experienced as incontinence and disorganization, and the propensity to act-out rather than verbalize). If one, on the other hand, conceptualizes transference as a special case of separate object-relations, and therefore makes pre-stages of transference synonymous with resistance against the transference, much conceptual and clinical obscurity is clarified. In this view, so-called psychotic and erotized transferences would be seen as resistances against the transference and not necessarily repetitions of past events. (The distinction I am drawing may reflect, from another viewpoint, the difference between miscellaneous "transferences" and the transference neurosis, proper.)

To the extent that transference phenomena are a refusal or inability to perceive the attributes of the current object faithfully but rather subjectively, it is a narcissistic phenomenon and constitutes resistance (against an object-relationship); to the extent that the preponderance of reactions are reality-oriented, and that perceptions and reactions from the past are used as a bridging function to a new and unique object, it is an object-directed (rather than self-directed) phenomenon: thus the dual nature of the transference. In this scheme, then, transference is a psychic function bridging both the narcissistic and object-related phases of development, still present in the neurotic and hopefully resolved at the completion of analysis with the achievement of full object-relatedness. That the capacity remains for re-analysis with its recrudescence of the transference reflects ever-present capacity for regression and/or persistence of narcissistic elements in healthy functioning. (A third possibility, that the development of the capacity for object-relations and transference is a cyclical rather than an aperiodic phenomenon, is a subject being treated separately.)

15   That narcissistic themes can be identified in later anal (obsessional) and phallic levels of functioning indicates that these conflicts and/or energies do not disappear from the psychic scene. In addition to the traditional repositories in the ego-ideal and in the ego-feeling (sense of self), character itself may represent the chief defense against an object-relationship, protecting against loss of identity and armoring the personality against invasion from the outside.

16   Altruistic and self-sufficient characters are often loosely referred to as narcissistic, and indeed may represent sublimations from this period; however, in many important respects they are the polar opposites of narcissists, an important clinical distinction.

17   In these terms, acting-out could be defined as the manipulation of another human being (doll-play) who has been imbued with the qualities necessary to a particular phantasy which is then enacted, the whole representing a one-sided (narcissistic) effort on the part of the actor to refuse to perceive the partner as a separate external being (resistance against an object-relationship, or transference) and to externalize and dramatize a phantasy (usually denying memory of actual experience).

When, however, the partner fails to comply and reacts, instead of to the phantasy, to the actors actual behavior (his denial of the partner's selfness, his projections and manipulation, the unreality of it all), a piece at least of a real object-relationship takes place, genuine object cathexis of the actor by the partner is felt, and the opportunity exists for friendly or therapeutic exploitation of the opening. This is the situation with narcissists in treatment. Acting with the patient in the misdirected hope of making "contact" not only destroys real contact and reproduces the traumatic effect of parental experience (annihilation of self), not only is it untherapeutic for the time, but creates grave barriers to the accessibility of the patient to subsequent efforts (iatrogenic damage), as well as sometimes having disastrous effects in the external life of the patient.

18   The free-floating attention, empathy, concern, helpfulness, and receptivity we carefully cultivate in analytic technique can and does become the target of the patient's manipulatory efforts, so much so that in some cases it becomes necessary to stop all interpretative work and at times even listening before the patient will begin to feel and think for himself (reminiscent of the conditions of children's' parallel play). In the case of Anne above, where mother did every task for her, any activity on the part of the analyst was misused at times as an occasion for her to be completely uninvolved herself.

19   The "tilt" described in the analytic situation with neurotics, the advantages accruing to the analyst which he must be careful not to abuse, in the case of narcissists is exactly the opposite, the analyst often finding it necessary to protect himself from being abused.

20   The narcissistic phase is resolved with the achievement of controlled bowel function, reflecting: (a) discharge of fused aggressive and libidinal energies to an unsplit object (ambivalence), (b) an autonomous act demonstrating ego (self) competence, toward itself and its object, and (c) satisfaction of id, ego, and superego simultaneously. It is a model of controlled, autonomous, socially responsible, constructive action and separate object-relatedness.

21   Historically, parents of narcissists, when signaled as needed, often did "take over" rather than collaborate, and trampled the "self", or oppositely, were so out of touch as to leave the child overwhelmed with internal stimuli which again functioned to destroy sense of self. In fact, rather than representing two reaction types, this alternation of attitudes is quite typical of narcissistic parents (whose object cathexis is limited and exercised only periodically) and accounts for the protracted binding to the parent; i.e., a uniformly rejecting or overprotective parent is easier to cope with.

22   This term is still used variously by different authors to denote three different entities, if used at all: as a modifier for "psychotic", as a wastebasket category, and as an abiding type of personality structure. It is used here in the latter sense, being synonymous with "narcissistic character". Perhaps it is that the underlying basis for this diagnostic category of borderline is more functional than pathognostic, representing those cases which lie outside the pale of our traditional techniques and thus injure our narcissism.

23 A word about prognosis: narcissistic patients always were difficult to treat, and I think they still are. The material presented here, while it has given me some feeling of understanding of these patients and some feeling of competence to deal with them, has been gathered more from clinical failure than success. I have only the conviction that after an encounter with such a patient, win-lose-or-draw, we both have learned something (if only that neither one of us is omnipotent).

24 If the narcissism is of significant proportions in the total clinical picture, attempts to analyze the overlaid neurotic accretions are not only useless but contribute to the resistance for later work, an iatrogenic aggravation often leading to eventual stalemate. These cases require that the character armor be analyzed first, though paradoxically, the patient may not permit it.

25 They will continually threaten to break off the treatment in an attempt to manipulate your concern. They may in fact do so, and the therapist must be prepared for it; any anxiety about losing the patient renders him lost already as a patient.

26 Some examples, the doses of which can be intensified as needed with the addition of humor and sarcasm: "You seem to want to be the analyst and have me the patient; I know you'd like to be my only patient, but we must stop now, I have another appointment; I am listening to you but I really don't know what you're talking about; are you perhaps trying to make me afraid of you; can you just tell me about it without making a production?; you seem to be aloof from all this that's going on; you seem to want to get everything you can without giving anything". Of course, a well-timed silence can be the most pointed remark of all.

27 No different in essence from the effect of any correct interpretation, which functions to "validate" a piece of the psyche from the inside and outside and thereby, by an increment, enlarge the "self".

"PITFALLS OF THERAPY"

By William S. Horowitz, M.D.

(Lecture at the Los Angeles Institute for Psychoanalysis
Extension Division
Course in Psychotherapy for Psychiatrists
October 30, 1961)

Ladies and Gentlemen:

I have chosen this topic rather than, say, "Brilliant Successes of Therapy", partly because it provides continuity with last week's discussion, but moreso because the actuality is that psychotherapy, as any medical or surgical procedure, entails risks and pitfalls both for the patient and the therapist; that this view is relatively neglected in our training programs; and that we, especially those of us in the formative stages of our careers, are prone to overlook these risks because of our almost universal occupational attitude (defense) of unwarranted therapeutic optimism or zeal.

Yes, I know, once in awhile we all see or are personally involved in a successful treatment situation which overcame enormous difficulties precisely because of the blind, naive, youthful ebullience of the therapist. I submit, however, that for every one of these gratifying exceptions there are five or ten or twenty miserable therapeutic failures entailing unnecessary discouragement to the patient and novice therapist, some of which are certainly avoidable. If we can understand and therefore anticipate the risks to come, we are in a better position, obviously, to avoid the avoidable.

If I have been impressed with any single consistent trait of older and therefore experienced psychotherapists, whatever their individual differences may be, it is the genuine caution and humility with which they undertake work with a new patient. Is this the fatigue of old age, or the sagacity of experience? I certainly do not intend to introduce a note of fear into our work, for I think there is already plenty of that in any therapist, especially one who is still clinging to omnipotence phantasies – but rather realistic caution.

It may have had a place once, early in medical school, to believe that a patient has his defenses and can't be damaged, or that a trainee only stands to learn from a failure experience – it may have helped all of us over our terror of facing alone another troubled human being and attempting to make sense of his illness and help him – but I submit that this pedagogical device or denial has outlived its usefulness and is a source of therapeutic ineffectiveness after the initial stages of training.

Eagerness not only leads to gross mistakes in patient and technique selection, but can drive away many sicker patients who would otherwise be quite workable. I think by now you have all come to appreciate the value and prognostic import of a patient approaching treatment with a healthy skepticism; I am only talking about its counterpart in the therapist. You know that the patient who dives right into therapy is a first cousin to the patient who doesn't come at all: do we find ourselves doing it?

I have some material here which was actually written up in another context and to illustrate another problem, namely contraindications to psychoanalysis, but which is largely applicable to our topic tonight and which can serve as a springboard for our discussion. To set the mood, so to speak, I want to read to you a poem taken from the Saturday Review of Literature of January 10th, 1959:

ON THE DEATH OF A STUDENT HOPELESSLY FAILING MY COURSE

By George Cuomo

He died the day before the last exam,
Leaving parents a lifetime of saying
"He could have made it, poor boy"

"Pitfalls Of Therapy"

> Poor boy, he
> could not. How little he could do in life!
> He lacked whole galaxies of talents, lacked
> quickness of hand or foot or eye or mind,
> Lacked will and ambition, lacked height and strength,
> Lacked even hope, lacked means of being hurt.
> He could swim well, he told me, and tried out,
> and did not make the team, and did not mind.
> Failure themed his small life, comforting him.
> He died racing a fire-red sports car,
> Soaring from the mountain roadway to spread
> a giant arc across the still night sky.

What position are we to take regarding this situation? Is the boy suffering from an "inferiority complex", a "failure neurosis"? Does the professor have something?... a healthy appreciation of the reality of the educational task and the boy's capacity? Is there something here for us? Should we speculate on the boy's early feeding, toilet and Oedipal experiences? Should we confirm the pertinence of these observations for the work of psychotherapy, too? Does a patient require the capacity to accomplish, does he need talents somewhere, does he need quickness of mind if not foot, does he need will and ambition, strength, hope, means of being hurt? Is there room, at least, for both points of view?

Can, or, should a psychotherapist be curious and sympathetic about the genesis and dynamics of an individual's problems, and make a realistic appraisal of his capacities at the same time? Further, does the therapist have a responsibility which the professor does not: to at least consider the possible relation between this particular failure experience and the ensuing suicide?

For a variety of reasons, people unsuitable for psychoanalysis or any kind of psychotherapy are presenting themselves with increasing frequency for treatment. For a variety of reasons the temptations are great to treat them, With the expansion of our art and science, and our actual increased capacity to be of help, the risk is present of attempting the impossible at no little cost to the patient, his family, the student analyst and the reputation of psychoanalysis in the community.

In treatment, we deal with a patient's ego. This is the agency which has proven inadequate for the patient and which brings him to us (usually), but it is also the tool with which we work. The clinician of a generation ago attempted to make an estimate of ego strength. Today, we are trying to refine just what that quality is, but its importance remains undiminished. I would go a step further. Before there were psychiatrists estimating ego strength, there were people estimating strength of character, of crucial importance in human relationships. The nub of my thesis is simply this – not every character is a character disorder or a treatable one.

I want to open for discussion the problems of ego strength and motivation. The issues of narcissism, quality of object relations, texture of superego, capacity of ego to bind instinct, utilize signal anxiety, think, sublimate, successfully defend, maintain friendly relations with reality, and so on, are all crucial to the success or failure of treatment. All this is commonplace, yet how often do we see in practice an indiscriminate, uniform, optimistic, uncovering, let's-see-how-far-the-patient-can-go approach. This error I think arises from two sources.

On the one hand, our skill at identifying bits of pathology far outstrips our knowledge of physiology. Of course, treatment of an isolated dynamic can be as foolish or as disastrous as in any other field of medicine. There is no patient in whom we cannot identify a relevant dynamic, but this has nothing to do with treatability of the whole patient, The novice psychotherapist and the experienced analyst who practices so-called "id analysis" commit the same fundamental error: mistaking identifying the deep pathology for treatment. It is the fallacy of the "successful" surgical operation with the patient, however, dying.

On the other hand, there is unresolved infantile omnipotence in the analyst which leads to unwarranted therapeutic optimism (or for that

"Pitfalls Of Therapy"

matter its opposite, an arrogant rejection of any but the most favorable patients). Both sources are at bottom one.

I would like to scan a few character "types" all of which I presume are familiar to you clinically and socially. At least, I hope they have wider circulation and relevance than to me alone. It's a peculiar thing, however. In my experience, cases of this kind are either passed off with, "Of course" or, "I never have experiences like that so I wouldn't know". I hope you will pardon this impressionistic approach. It is understood that these qualities actually represent quantitative relations not measurable at present, and therefore assessed by clinical judgment. I hope the discussion will bring out the internal economic situation which mitigates for or against successful treatments as well as the numerous other examples I am sure exist.

I do not present these as absolute contraindications to treatment but rather problems which must be apprehended immediately if grief is to be spared. As you see, I leave to one side the question of classification and those cases very familiar to you from the literature. I want to bring up what is not often written about nor talked about. One eventuality I would anticipate in our discussion to follow is that of a moral tone entering, followed by a reactive democratic protest; the counterparts of the therapeutic pessimism and optimism referred to before. I think such attitudes would be as totally out of place as, for instance, would be the following sentiment: "All congenital heart patients ought to be given the benefit of the latest surgical procedure for correction of their lesions, for after all, their life and productiveness is at stake". The failure to assess suitability for this particular procedure would be obvious. Again I repeat, in treatment we deal with the patient's ego.

Now for some illustrations:

The contemptuous, lacking a sense of decency and respect for people. Eleanor, a 42 year old woman, comes for advice on how to get rid of her husband of some 20 years. She says, "And I wouldn't be seeing you, either,

"Pitfalls Of Therapy"

if I had to spend my own money", of which she has a goodly amount. "I have a policy that pays," she says, "Charge the company whatever you like!"

The dishonest, unable to enter into a trustworthy treatment compact. Norman, a 37 year old artist, places an emergency call from a phone booth near his home, claiming that his wife needs to be seen immediately, and that he was referred by an internist who, indeed, is familiar to me. He pauses to bargain over the phone, will I accept paintings in lieu of money for treatment? "They will be eventually much more valuable." His wife proves to have a lifelong character problem and avers she has had no treatment for it. A call to the internist reveals that she has just left one of my colleagues and that, further, litigation is pending over a minor physical injury which they hope will solve all their financial problems.

The castrator, not limited to women, but including some impotent men whose dominating unconscious aim is to render the therapist helpless, the gratification of which supersedes all else. Seductiveness, immediate crushes on the therapist, chumminess, patronizing indulgence of him, or hypocritical sincerity, can all mask this aim. Frances, a 37 year old divorced woman, comes for psychiatric treatment, concomitantly with starting a course of dancing lessons and signing up with a marriage broker. "It can't hurt, can it?" She professes the therapist is just the man she is looking for, won't he tell her about his personal life, too? Of course, she knows she can't expect a social relationship from him, or can she? So, what has he to offer?

The mouth, or yawning abyss, the patient who wants from the very beginning and doesn't hesitate to demand. He must be rapidly confronted with the question of what he is willing to give. Marvin, a 30 year old psychiatric case worker, applies to the Clinic with the understanding it is there to provide an easy analysis to some people. Shocked that he will be charged for initial interviews, he brightens with the idea, "Well, if I'm accepted for analysis, then my wife will have to go to work."

The postponer, eager for and serious about treatment but not now. Ted, an 18 year old student, makes a good impression on the Clinic

"Pitfalls Of Therapy"

admissions committee and, after acceptance, convinces them what a good case he is by periodic calls over a year's time expressing his continued interest. When called to start, he states he is thrilled and ready, but would the therapist be willing to wait three months because he has such a good summer job?

The success, the patient who is too successful and gratified in his personal life, to which he can flee at the first storm signal. Bill, a 27 year old Ph.D. in metallurgy, president of his professional society, university instructor, author, businessman, and quite facile with the ladies, comes for help to free himself from a current love affair which he recognizes is self-destructive and in the pattern of his unsuccessful marriage. In short order this is accomplished in psychotherapy and he plunges into analysis to clear up everything, including his troublesome manifest homosexuality. Thirty-five hours later, he smilingly announces one Monday morning that he won a new bride in Las Vegas the night before and his analysis will have to wait for the future.

The make-believe, the fake or phony character, the empty character, the mannequin, the stereotype, the embodiment of a retail advertisement who speaks exclusively in clichés. Laurel, a 19 year old dental technician, attired in the latest Beverly Hills chic uniform, wore unusually peaked painted eyebrows, on which obviously more attention had been lavished each morning than what she described her infant son received. She silently invited me to open doors for her and light her cigarette with svelte gestures and postures, any one of which if caught in midair by high speed photography I'm sure she hoped would win her a page in a fashion magazine, everlasting fame, the hand of the boss, and so on. Her problem was that mother disapproved of her dating a fellow of another faith.

The shoppers who treats selecting a therapist like pinching fruit. Our friend Frances again called a series of therapists on the telephone, nonplused at some of the exasperated responses she elicited when she inquired of each of them his marital status, the number of issue the union bore, as well as perhaps did they play golf? Each of these crucial facts had their own personal meaning to her, needless to say, and her relentless search was only temporarily slowed by my naive attempt to contact her.

The chronic patient, already through a succession of therapists over a 5 to 15 year period, smilingly or gamely ready to start afresh. Treatment has become a way of life, familiar to us from other branches of medicine. Jane, a middle-aged psychiatric case worker, presents herself for therapy, unduly optimistically considering a several-year analysis with an excellent senior analyst, a period of psychotherapy with the same man, and another period with another therapist, the whole stretching back about 10 years. She complains that they had done nothing for her, but is ready to start in again, undaunted.

One can be certain in such a case that, aside from the issues of unconscious sense of guilt, masochism, etc, the patient has succeeded in a re-enactment of one or several unconscious fantasies with her therapist. I think here one must be especially acute to conditions the patient lays down for her therapy, no matter how well they seem to be grounded in rational necessity, for it is in the arrangements about time and money, I feel, that the unseen defense and gratification is to be found.

The bizarre, who, in the presence of seemingly good functioning, tolerates extremely peculiar ego contortions. Actually, of course, these people are extremely disturbed and able to function only because of these circumscribed ego deformities. Naomi, a 25 year old woman of very high intelligence, is in jeopardy of losing her well-paid job in theoretical mathematics and computer programming because she can't get to work on time. The problem is that she never knows what time it is, for she doesn't wear a watch. Later, among other things, it emerges that she sleeps in the same room with her brother and keeps her clothes in a suitcase, berating her parents all the while for not providing more adequate quarters.

The amorphous, the patient without identity or structure. It is often impossible for them to distinguish an instinctual urge, from an ego judgment, from a superego command, from a drive emanating from another individual entirely. Closely related are the infantilized or spoiled and the symbiotic.

There are, obviously, many other types — the reasonable patient usually intellectually controlling a most unreasonable sadism; the normal asymptomatic, unmotivated patient presenting himself for a variety of reasons, excluding being sick; the denier; the con man; the litigious type; the pitiful one to be rescued, which is one of a variety of fantasies a patient may appeal to you to re-enact with him; the controller, who immediately sets conditions to the treatment; the patient who wants you only to intercede in his reality; and the patient who puts up a continuous pressure for you to change your methods of operation.

Cecilia, a 29 year old mathematician, presented an unusually rich combination of such "challenges", She came to the Psychoanalytic Clinic not with a complaint but a formulation: namely, she supposed that she suffered from a father transference to men which compelled her to sleep with them, although it later proved that this had happened only twice. She indicated that she had deferred all of her problems until the day she could be analyzed. She made her plans in terms of a 6-month's period of treatment. It is interesting and I think significant that each of 5 interviewers saw a distinct facet of her personality.

On entering the consultation room, she complimented the analyst on his alma mater. At the end of the hour, she demanded an immediate decision as to her acceptability. A portion of her story was that she worked at the same industrial plant as her husband but was disgruntled that she was not afforded the same recognition as he because of her lack of a degree. She told how she had either fought with or seduced her various bosses. She could not stand her child but wanted to become pregnant again because she felt so good then. Security regulations prevented her from discussing certain things.

It was further revealed that the family income was substantial enough to provide private psychotherapy for both marital partners, not to mention the existence of a major medical policy. It turned out that she lived under an assumed name and identity in adolescence for four years, ostensibly in order to support her family. An interesting arrangement in her current household was that the family home remained unlocked during the day when all three members were away, but was locked at night when she retired to bed with her daughter. The husband, who came home later, had no key and each evening pounded on the door to be admitted.

Failure is not always a product of neurotic need-to-fail, (there is really such a thing as inadequacy), and yet, how often in overlooking this obvious point do we belie our own infantile idea that to name it is to conquer it. We all, at one time, on discovering psychoanalysis, experienced the promise of universal cure. How easily we forget the difficult achievements of our own analysis and are willing to subject a patient who has never achieved anything to the same procedure. I remind you again of the poem with which we started.

Now I'd like to try to focus down, after these descriptive remarks, on the issues which I think are elemental to this discussion. As I view it, the pitfall of psychotherapy is the perversion of what ought to be a doctor-patient therapeutic relationship into an acting-out untherapeutic relationship. What is meant by this? Acting-out refers to a dramatization, an enactment, a staging taking place between two people. It entails one partner, the active initiator, struggling with some memory of past painful experience and its covering and denying phantasy which is entirely forgotten and unconscious, seducing another person, the passive, willing and unwitting partner, into playing a role with him, the purpose of which is to live out this phantasy and still maintain the denied experience in unawareness.

In this, the quality of action is predominant over speech, although specific "lines" to be spoken may play a crucial part. The action gives itself away by its inappropriateness to the reality circumstance at hand (though the initiator will defend its reasonableness to the bitter end), and by the passive partner's perception, if he is sensitive, that he is being used for something, that a phantasied image of himself is being seen by the other rather than his real self.

We might tabulate this as follows: acting-out involves:

1) Lack of contact with current and past reality.
2) A false or pseudo-object-relationship in which any object will do.
3) A repressed painful memory and unconscious denying phantasy.
4) A regressed state of ego-functioning in which action replaces ideation, the compulsion to repeat is paramount, and mastery is directed at the past.
5) The total projection of the unconscious material (objects, experience, affects and impulses, and denying phantasy) onto the current reality situation, with attempts to manipulate it to fit or "play".

Transference, per se, is obviously a related phenomenon, but has these differences: the initiator has some perspective; he can see (potentially) simultaneously his projection and can grasp the reality of the other person ("It's amazing how angry I get when you use that tone of voice, it's exactly like my father, and yet I know you're not"); the other person is used in a different way, is needed as a concrete specific object on which to hang a piece of repressed content in order to deal with it and the new person.

We might tabulate this as follows: transference involves:

1) Good contact with current and past reality.
2) A real object-relationship present and past, the present object selected and meaningful partly because remindful of past object.
3) Repressed unconscious material not necessarily highly conflictual and pressing for emergence.
4) An unregressed state of ego-functioning, in which adaptation to and mastery of current reality paramount, conservation of the meaningful object-relationship important, action replaced by affects and thinking, repetition of the old superseded by discovery of the new and different.

5) A projection of only a piece of the old object, usually a single physical or mental attribute, and a displacement of usually only a predominant affect from the old to the current object. The aim is not exclusively mastery of the undigested old object but just as important is the bridging function from the mastered and familiar old to the desired and unknown new.

You can see immediately how much more propitious this state of affairs is for therapy, since the patient has a healthy grasp of the external reality and object, has a real object-relationship with you, has a dawning awareness of a something from his unconscious and past emerging, and works with it rather than playing with it. I don't have to remind you that just as a patient can transfer (displace and rediscover) onto his therapist, so the therapist can transfer onto his patient attitudes toward significant specific objects in his past. Likewise, just as the patient can try to engage the therapist in acting-out some unconscious phantasy from childhood, so the therapist can try to involve the patient in the same thing relative to his own past.

To be distinguished from transference (and counter-transference) and acting-out (and counter-acting-out) is a third transaction: what we can call, for lack of a better term, reacting. I use this term to denote having feelings or impulses to action based on realistic considerations rather than on one's own past history: having responses which probably anyone might have in any kind of situation, social or therapeutic, although how the response is expressed, how it is discharged, might be quite different in the two situations.

These reactions are, by and large, based on the normal economy and regulation of healthy narcissism (self-esteem) and reality-testing. If a patient literally steps on your toes, it hurts and offends, and you are angry; this is reacting and it is normal. If you should then knee him in the groin in retaliation, then that would be over-reacting, another matter. It is very easy, sometimes, in the relaxed, intimate, and sympathetic atmosphere of the psychotherapy situation, for the therapist to regress right along with his patient and either feel ashamed of and inhibit his normal reactions, or feel licensed to over-react as he might not even in an ordinary social setting. He may be tempted also, in this setting, to be ashamed of his counter-transferences and avoid working with them internally (a very fruitful source of help for the treatment), or, may feel licensed to act upon them. Thirdly, of course, he may accept his patient's invitation to tango, or offer his own brand of acting-out. As you see, the villain throughout is acting.

Can we list then some of the signals by which a therapist may begin to suspect he is experiencing a counter-transference reaction, if he is not immediately aware of it?

1) Usually involves a single patient, or at most, a single type or class of patients.
2) Undue affects: liking or disliking the patient beyond the usual range of feeling toward other patients.
3) Instinctual discharges toward patient: actual sexual excitement or felt rage.
4) Undue preoccupation with patient after hours, phantasies, appearance of the patient in the therapist's dreams.
5) Under- or over-estimation of the patient's capacities, or unusual obscurity in understanding the patient's diagnosis, dynamics, or emerging material (especially when not shared by colleagues).
6) Willingness to make very unusual arrangements for the patient.

These, then, and other signs may signal that a particular patient has become the carrier of particular attributes of a significant object in the therapist's past and the target, then, of irrational and inappropriate affects and urges. This phenomenon is usually found in the context of otherwise good functioning, as we have noted, occurs not infrequently, and is eminently workable.

In distinction to this, when a therapist is engaged in acting-out, it usually involves all his patients, in one form or another, and his family, friends, and colleagues as well (any object will do). What is acted-out is usually something infantile, usually something embedded in the therapist's character, and usually rooted in his narcissism (belied by his using people to stage something from within, filling his needs and not theirs). This phenomenon is more regressive, much harder for the therapist to grasp and work with, but by the same token, much more important and fruitful to work with. For our purposes tonight, we can round this out by making over-reactions and acted-upon counter-transferences synonymous with acting-out.

Some sample acted-out phantasies or results of them:

Narcissistic level: using patients as a source of narcissistic supplies, rather than outside life.

1) Driving ambition to have them succeed, or fail.
2) As audience for private views, to carry out private missions.
3) Need to seduce and be liked, be popular.
4) Infantilizing.
5) Irritability over psychotherapy work, feeling imposed on by patients, feeling impatient over the interruption of more important academic, administrative, or scientific activities.
6) Acting the savior, martyr, messiah, prophet, prodigal son, son of God, or God himself.
7) Pygmalion, Galatea, silk-purse making.

Oral

1) Feeding patients too much, or waiting to be fed by them.
2) Over-empathizing, identifying.
3) Inability to terminate treatment.

Anal

1) Exploiting patients (professionally, money, time).
2) Making treatment a torture for the patients, attacking, etc.

3) Allowing self to be tortured by patients, allowing then, to become your persecutors.

Phallic. and Oedipal

1) Rescuing.
2) Manipulating wife against husband, vice versa, child vs. parent.

To step back now and take perspective, we can see that just as the patient's defense mechanisms against his unconscious, in the treatment situation become directed against the therapist and constitute his resistance – so the therapist's defenses against his unconscious become, in the treatment situation, directed against the patient and constitute his resistance. You will indulge me, I trust, if I make the following sweeping generalization: the resistance of the student therapist is his infantile narcissism, the defense against feelings of helplessness.

When the defense is working at full steam, it manifests itself in phantasies of omnipotence and omniscience, and feelings of arrogance and unwarranted therapeutic optimism or zeal. When the defense is not working so effectively, then we see the underlying helpless attitude emerging, which manifests itself in the other ubiquitous problem of young therapists: identifying with the patient's defenses, identifying with the patient, becoming, as it were, in his shoes.

When, of course, the therapist has learned enough technique to be confident of his real ability to help, and has undergone maturation in the meanwhile, he has no further need for these defenses and assumes his rightful place in the therapeutic setting: neither God nor the patient, but the helper with something real to offer.

We all understand that this is no slur on our professional escutcheons. It is only a membership card in the human race, documenting that all of us were once children and felt helpless, that we all struggled with this impossible feeling by erecting phantasies of how powerful we were, and that these attitudes were corrected in the course of time, only to be revived and worked through again each time we started in a new stage of our lives and careers. The only slur, or better, sickness, is if these troubles do not get corrected in the course of training and experience; then, of course, we will be wise enough to know how to get help.

SEXUAL ADDICTION

After viewing the ABC special on this subject (1/24/97), reading a bit into Carnes' book detailing his invention of the topic, and being exposed to mass-treatment of offenders by "group-therapy", I am compelled to sort out the many conceptualizations rivalling for attention in my head.

The proponents of this diagnostic perspective seem to eagerly and indiscriminately include all types of aberrant behavior, regardless of instinctual object, aim, or implementation into the rubric of addiction. We could call it a rubber rubric for its elasticity. And the treatment approach is always the same: place disparate people and syndromes willy-nilly into 12-step programs of group therapy in which the goal is to reach "sobriety". The end-goal is acknowledged to be unattainable and require life-long working of "the program", for the "addict" is never free of his propensity for addiction. What is clear is that the subject is never free of treatment, paying a nominal price to the therapist to exorcise and control his waywardness, not unlike the leverage some religions practice to capture their flock: first, damn them as sinners, then invite them in for redemption.

My conception of addiction is a failure to develop beyond an early oral fixation on achieving a fusion experience with mother, the etiology often being her rejection of the subject. The intoxicated state can achieve this early fusion experience with the world, so seductive as to be repetitiously and monotonously sought throughout life, superceding any other goals and effectively preventing further development. To the extent that the group, its leader, or the subject's sponsor can serve as supporting and nurturing surrogates for mother, and to the extent that the procedures enhance taking responsibility for one's own actions (and therefore supporting ego and superego development and delivering some sense of self-control), I can understand how AA can have some effect on substance abusers, imperfect as it may be.

On the other hand, the patients I have worked with who have suffered with the symptom of compulsive sexual activity accompanied by obsessional preoccupation with it, seem to have an entirely different etiology. It is well-known that these patients more often than not had been the victims of sexual abuse in their childhood. The effect of overtly sexual stimulation on a young child, as is the effect of overtly violent victimization, is to flood the immature organism with excitation. The over-stimulation cannot be discharged because channels for discharge have yet to be developed; because it cannot be conceptualized because of the child's immature comprehension; because the child can only passively experience it at the time. The result is the overwhelmed state we call traumatic.

This early pathologic state of psychic economy results in massive inchoate explosions of affect, dread of the arising of any inner sensation, mistrust and withdrawal from the world, and attempts to master the passively-experienced overwhelmed state by converting passive into active, doing to others what has been done to him. Characteristic of the economic state of affairs, the massive over-excitation is quantitatively so preponderant over the child's ability to discharge it that the trauma is repetively experienced and re-worked almost daily, in dreams which often awaken into nightmares, and in obsessional preoccupation with the themes. This repetitious re-working of the trauma is the attempt by the subject to master or overcome the traumatized state, and is what distinguishes it from the object-seeking union with the primal object in addiction.

So-called "sexual addicts" display this pathognomonic behavior of fear of the arising of impulses and the need to discharge them immediately and indiscriminately before they can assume overwhelming proportions. This struggle for self-control may resemble the true addict's fight against his cravings, but is fundamentally different. The addict is struggling to control his urge for something which has pleasurable connotations; the traumatized one is struggling against mounting arousal which has unpleasant connotations. So, the true addict is object- and sensation-seeking; the traumatic neurotic is sensation-avoiding.

Both are characterized by repetitious behavior, but then again, so are most sufferers from psychological disorders. Both are often chronic and intractable. Both are the products of inadequate parenting. Both often lead to anti-social and self-destructive acts and law-breaking. Both often come to the attention of the mental health professional via the courts. And perhaps a particular case needn't be a pure example but have admixtures of both states. But it still seems important to distinguish the etiology and pathology of these states in planning a rational treatment approach, regardless of one's theoretical orientation.

DOES THE PATIENT HAVE TO WORK ?

William S. Horowitz, M.D.

March 23, 2005

Musing on the problem of an interminable psychoanalysis, although conducted with standard then modified technique with an above-average talented and intelligent patient, I found myself wondering about the absence of effectuality in his existential life as well as within the treatment, where he manifested high expectations, facile regurgitation of interpretations and insights, borrowing and exploiting the accomplishments of others, jackrabbit changes of course in life, and inability to stand on his own or achieve satisfaction.

He was the youngest of three living children of immigrant parents, separated from his next sibling by 15 years, essentially an only child in his family, indulged by his pretentious mother and nursed for 2 years; a childhood bed-wetter of bright intelligence and a quick student who never-theless complained that he needed the analyst's help well past adulthood for a variety of difficulties which he never seemed to learn about and overcome. His relations with his objects could be described as parasitic: taking what he needed, leaving his detritus.

He was obviously well-read and interested in a variety of topics in his world view, and thus able to converse on a high level and impress listeners with his knowledge, grasp of issues, and assemble convincing arguments in his fascinating writings, giving the impression of an original and highly intelligent mind. However, he complained that he could not choose between his variegated career interests, and exhibited a certain capriciousness in his preoccupations of the moment and his various human relationships. He could be described as a dilettante of some depth.

Work-Does The Patient Have To Work?

He had many of the stigmata of A.D.D. including impulsivity, restlessness, inability to focus, difficulty reading and taking in, inability to learn, and the pathognomonic paradoxical reaction to stimulants, with which he experimented throughout his life with little apparent lasting benefit.

As a rule, he responded with keen interest to my interventions, and was able to elaborate the idea in a rich profusion of associations with the conviction that the insight was indeed meaningful...but, nothing stuck! An interesting ancillary observation was a long pause after my interpretations, longer than is usual with others, perhaps betokening a resistance at work. It was all intellectual: fascinating and seductive, but lacking permanence. Only after years of trying to help him bring his treatment to a satisfactory closure did I experience exasperation with the repetitive task and no lasting results, finally associating the thought that he got straight A's in school without ever studying!! This was to me a thunderbolt which solidified my conviction that finally we were on the right track.

What was missing, I came to believe, was the process of "working through", the repetitive confronting of relevant issues of impulse v. defense in a current and historical perspective, with the consequent incorporation of the solution into abiding structure, i.e. genuine learning or the laying down of permanent neurological pathways or psychological convictions. Each moiety of learning, achievement of a mental skill, ratifies and enlarges the self and contributes a sense of agency to it. "It is not just happening, is not happening to me, I am doing it."

What was missing was the felt necessity to *work* for what he wanted, to expend effort, repeatedly, until his ability to gain satisfaction was won, the achievement of a skill, for apparently in his mind everything would come to him as if by magic. It is indeed a variety of magical thinking that to name it, to say it, was the equivalent of knowing it, possessing it, having it; thus the facile use of ideas and language but the inability to navigate in the real world of hard facts to garner what he desired and achieve satisfaction. These patients have the unconscious phantasy that the analyst will deliver the magical words and insights that will cure their problem and bring them satisfaction; that analysis is a magical procedure. Perhaps they are not alone in this idea.

This expected magical arrival of what is desired, like hallucinatory wish-fulfillment, is not only the product of immaturity, nor yet of parental undue gratification, but also of the high intelligence to which ideas "just come" out of nowhere. These creative individuals are the passive recipients of their Muse, but then the idea must be worked upon and elaborated in an artistic or inventive fashion if it is not to result in mere smearing. This elaboration requires work, too: the well-known "perspiration" after the "inspiration". (In physics, the formula for work is energy expended through distance.)

A second patient comes to mind, a man with again a very high intelligence and signs of A.D.D. who accomplished important and impressive achievements in his chosen scientific field but who was so emotionally unstable that he could not sustain a workmanlike development of his inventions and techniques, (ones which impressed older professionals around him), but collapsed almost like a sand-castle which implodes upon itself when it reaches undue height. He, too, was an autodidact, who took minimal insights from his treatment to process them himself in seclusion rather than in collaboration. He had been a precocious little nursery student with two parents almost totally unable to communicate meaningfully with him.

We usually think of working-through as a *minor* accompaniment to the process of incorporation and digestion of the analysis, a product of the repetition-compulsion and the necessity to confront issues repeatedly, possibly on successively higher levels. In these patients, however, it seems to be the *central* issue in their failure to grow and complete their analyses. Specifically because they were and are bright, they never developed habits of expending effort in a sustained fashion to get what they wanted, to work at it, until possession of skills to achieve gratification and incorporate structure was accomplished. They play at life.

I found it necessary to explicitly stop the "treatment", which was endlessly gratifying and thus not growth-promoting, and assume instead the role of mentor, coach, or good parent. Withholding the "therapeutic" non-judgmental, ever-available, understanding, and dispensing of all-seeing comments and substituting instead much rarer contacts along the lines of "counseling" seemed to have a salutary effect, especially as it resulted in a heightened frustration for him and the passing of responsibility for the achievement of relief from me to him. He did not experience this as abandonment, although initially he was shocked by it, until he realized I was still available for occasional guidance while he grew his sea legs. The formal treatment was over, the "relationship therapy" (concept of Maurice Levine, M.D., Cincinnati) was in operation, he had been weaned.

This is but an example of the general problem of the narcissistic gratification in the treatment situation that is usually unperceived and which is the greatest factor in the common failure to effect a "cure", I believe. It is, in this perspective, iatrogenic. (See my paper on "Narcissism"). Patients seek the "perfect parent" to cure their historical troubles, and we unthinkingly fall into gratifying that phantasy by our extended and intensive techniques. Don't blame Freud. He usually treated for *months* and not intensively; we in the U.S. treat daily for *years*. Americans are fat and overindulged; do we parents tend to spoil them?

POSTSCRIPT

I cannot conclude this collection without mentioning my retrospective opinion about the psychoanalytic technique I was taught. The American classical approach, "improved and perfected" from the original experimental attempts of the Master, carries with it an unadvertised side effect of undue gratification, stemming from the patient having the analyst's attention and concern in unlimited amounts. This narcissistic bonus may account for many "interminable" analyses, which I doubt plagued Freud who treated for months, not years.

LET MY PEOPLE GO!:
AN ESSAY ON JEWISH ATAVISM AND THEOCRACY.

William S. Horowitz, M.D.

Dedicated to my son and the spirit of my father.

I propose this paper as a so-called "thought experiment" in psycho-ethnology, not as a full exegesis of an hypothesis, but as an essay to encourage reflection, discussion, and scholarly research by others better equipped for that task. I make no apology for this abbreviation, offering it as a worthwhile thesis for consideration never-the-less. Having no pretensions to authoring the *last* word, my aim will be accomplished if this sometimes abrupt *first* word breaks the social taboo and starts such a process going.

The source of my material has been the clinical psychoanalytic situation, working with patients for now over four decades, in addition to having been living in the society and observing it, and myself, from the same point of view: what is going on in the unconscious? Freud compared psycho-analysis to archeology, the reconstruction of what may or must have been from buried fragments, and *this* constitutes the unique contribution of the psychoanalyst, distinctive from all other sources but of course requiring confirmation or refutation from those other sources.

Those readers unaccustomed to working with depth psychology, unschooled in the basic biological sciences, or holding devout religious convictions (not to mention those who simply disagree), will expectably experience strong resistance to these ideas, which is a regrettable loss of audience but a problem which is not mine to address, particularly in this brief declarative schema. But, given the gravity of the subject matter, even the skeptics may feel compelled to give this thesis consideration: between the twin assaults of extermination and assimilation, the homo sapiens judaicus may well constitute an endangered species.

Let My People Go!: An Essay On Jewish Atavism And Theocracy.

I have no intention of an attack on a people nor a religion *per se* which should compel defensiveness and the reiteration of dogma, for a thoughtful reading of this paper will reveal my affirming and conserving aim: to attack analytically and resolve the *capture* of both of them, the people and the religion, by fixating anti-developmental forces. The intention is "therapeutic," the hope that the understanding of these historical and psychological experiences can result in the freeing up and resumption of growth and renewal in the group.

It should be noted at the outset that when referring to Jews in the following text, I have in mind the portrait of the Jew in classical literature, the European *Ostjuden*, or the Hasidic Jew in contemporary American society as exemplars of what I am describing, rather than the socially-assimilated Western-dressed and -mannered Jew, member of the world community. However, it will be quickly realized that the former only serve to demonstrate by exaggeration many traits of the latter.

Merchant of Venice, I,iii,111, Shylock: "...For sufferance is the badge of all our tribe. You call me misbeliever, cut-throat dog, and spit upon my Jewish gaberdine, and all for use of that which is mine own."

To the argument that the range of attributes or behaviors between individuals in this or any group exceeds the differences between groups and therefore makes characterizations of groups impossible, I would offer that the very word *group* already denotes commonalities amongst its members. We have a long and respected tradition in biology and medicine of collating descriptive and functional attributes in our *taxonomy*, disparate symptoms into *syndromes*, and behavioral clusters into *developmental levels*, without being questioned about its "unfairness". Obviously, emotions (narcissism) and politics (power relationships) come into play when attempting to describe national, religious, or political clusters of attributes, which may be just as self-evident as any other group characteristic but which may induce the defenses of denial and *scotomata* from the above sources, and from the peculiarly American prohibition against making discriminations. The possibility (and history) of *abuse* of objective observation should make us careful, to be sure, but not blind.

Let My People Go!: An Essay On Jewish Atavism And Theocracy.

I

On viewing the soaring vaults of the nave of the Santa Maria Novella in Florence, it suddenly came to me that the Jews are non-believers: skeptics, apostates, cynics, paranoids. Not just of the divinity of Christ; they refuse to believe, period. In the religious architecture, it is rationalized as not believing in heaven, hence no upward pointing artifacts. But in fact, there is no upward pointing anything, no elevation of the spirit, no belief in anything higher, including and most importantly their own better selves. Underneath, they see themselves as abandoned, alone, and accursed, an obvious, it seems to me, incorporation of their former slave status.

They believe in a God, it will be pointed out, but curiously and significantly even He is not elevated, *nor even represented*. Many religions have their clergy dressed in robes, shawls, and ceremonial headdresses, but most uncover (or show other signs of obeisance such as bending the knee) when addressing their Lord in prayer. Not so the orthodox Jew, who keeps his *secular* fedora on along with his congregation, ala a "committee of the whole" *without a lord in attendance.*

There may be a dual inference here: on the one hand this may reflect the worshiper's feeling of abandonment by his God and the necessity to carry on alone, and on the other, that the abandoning God is not needed, that the subject can be the god himself. This renders the (confusing) picture of his omnipotence overlaying his impotence, both of which function as strong provocations to those who do not share his (dis) belief in himself. Both aspects are reflected again in his posing as the authority/buttressing his sagging sense of masculinity by wearing his hat and beard, as he forcibly segregates the women and keeps a Sabbath "Goy" at home and the synagogue to do his menial work, a likely repetition of what the overlords did to him. Peter Gay (1987) quotes Freud's self-designation as a "completely Godless Jew" in spite of being proudly ethnically identified, raising the question to what degree he may be reflective of a trend amongst Jews in general.

Let My People Go!: An Essay On Jewish Atavism And Theocracy.

Judaism is a psychology of the slave, I postulate, perpetuated in part by the annual reminder, nay *celebration*, of the Jews' historical role in bondage and struggle for freedom (always against an outer tyrant, of course). They latently hate themselves and behave in such a way as to embody that self-hatred, then project that self-hatred onto external "anti-Semites" and provoke attack from them: by that projection, by their "difference", by their asserted superiority, and by that transparent embodiment of some of the most shameful of human traits...just as a derelict, rejected by his family and then society, lies in the street and draws the contempt and perhaps kicks of those standing (...and just as a depressed patient, rejected by his unbearably harsh super-ego, projects that super-ego into a hateful environment and proceeds to elicit condemnation from it).

Not only is the slave required to do the dirty work of the society, but he is used as a repository for all the disavowed and projected unacceptable psychic contents of the society, thereby rendering him both a garbage collector and a garbage dump. *This* is the chief source of the self-loathing of the slave.

In addition, as if this were not enough, those who have experienced the underclass in a society, viewing that society from beneath the heel of a master, undergo a powerful process of disillusionment which makes it impossible to entertain the phantasy of the "good life" they once shared as free men with the rest of that society, accounting for the dis-belief or cynicism we are struck by in populations which reside in or have emerged from the underclass: viz., slaves, criminals, abandoned children, etc. This loss of the capacity to re-believe, to share in one of the necessary delusions of life (another being the denial of death), is an enduring psychological state which is not readily overcome, and which acts as a further irritating reminder to the rest of society provoking in it guilt, defensiveness, and sometimes counter-attacks.

Anti-Semitism is a perfectly rational reaction by Jews and non-Jews alike, in this thesis, to the *unconscious* defeated and denigrated qualities in the classic Jewish culture which are vigorously repressed, denied, and dignified into their opposites or externalized, after which an attempt is made to salvage some modicum of self-respect and consolation from the lore, history, and glorified reaction-formations.

Mer. of Ven., V,i,69, Jessica: "I am never merry when I hear sweet music." V,i,83, Lorenzo: "The man that hath no music in himself, nor is not moved with concord of sweet sounds, is fit for treasons, stratagems and spoils; the motions of his spirit are dull as night and his affections dark as Erebus: let no such man be trusted."

The traditional secular music of the Jews is minor key and sad (lamentation), the pictures tortured, the literature introspective, the architecture un-lofty, the dress black, the language un-euphonious. There is an undeniable absence of an esthetic here which goes much deeper than the "prohibition against graven images", lying in a lack of harmony within, in my opinion. The Jew is simply not at peace within himself and with his world and his God. There is no joyousness or bliss. The soul of the Jew is unhappy.

However, I would sharply distinguish between actual anti-Semitism, i.e. external reactions to perceived provocative qualities in the culture, from the institutionalized automatic expectation of it *by* Jews, which is the construction of an abiding external (interchangeable) enemy arising from, causing, and justifying paranoid anxieties and the discounting of criticism in general, both products of narcissistic operations. ("You criticize because you hate me.") Not to be overlooked is the use of the accusation of anti-Semitism as an easy "justified" attack on the "perpetrator" which is laboriously difficult to rebut, relatively risk-free to the accuser, and more often than not effective in manipulating the imputed guilty party into silence; most parents undoubtedly have experienced this "ploy" from their children.

There is also the possibility of anti-Semitism arising from independent external sources, of course, but it is striking to realize that of all the religions, nationalities and cultures, *this* anti- alone has become reified.

There is a *biologically*-based automatic antipathy toward the *other* species or races of man which works against miscegenation, underscored by

Let My People Go!: An Essay On Jewish Atavism And Theocracy.

Sheldon's finding (1944) that spouses tend to find partners of similar skull (and facial) size and configuration. This would tend to explain ingrained social repulsion between the races, but not anti-Semitism which is not racial. But anthropologically and sociologically speaking, there is well-known *tribal* rivalry which tends to segregate human groups into distinctive in-bred cultures, corresponding on a group level to the individual's secondary narcissistic effort to delineate his "self", and *this*, I believe, most closely approximates the phenomenon of anti-Semitism. This view of anti-Semitism would universalize the phenomenon and rob it of its uniqueness and therefore rationale for special treatment. This would say to the aggrieved Jew, "So, everyone doesn't love you...so what? Is it any different for anyone else?"

It is the enforced bondage of one generation to the next, and of the individual to his "faith" or "people" which is the operant incorporated psychic slavery, the perpetuation of the external historical fact.

Physical enslavement was not limited to ancient Egypt by any means; modern history continues the "tradition" by social and occupational ghettoization in almost all societies and eras, of which perhaps the most extreme examples took place in this century during WWII. When I hear amongst Westernized Jews the praises sung of Jewish "tradition", it is *this* tradition which comes to mind.

Freud (1939) postulates that the Jewish religion was *imposed* on the Hebrew tribes by Moses the Egyptian, though he curiously makes no mention of their slave status, nor their likely blackness. Paul Johnson (1988) makes multiple references to the forced imposition of labor and religious belief on the Hebrew tribes when enslaved, and by them in turn when they enslaved others. The historical fact of this behavior proves the incorporation of what was done to them, what we know as identification with the aggressor, suggesting that this incorporated slave-master resided somewhere in their ego and/or its superstructures and thus may have extended to the conception of their god. With little doubt, the *coercion* is reflected in the religion.

Let My People Go!: An Essay On Jewish Atavism And Theocracy.

Where, for example, in charitable fund-raising practice, never an encouraging word is heard, such as *please* and *thank you*. More consequentially, the sentiment is often voiced, "Once a Jew, always a Jew". Catholics and Protestants shift into, out of, and between various denominations and ministries with no such sentiment expressed. The *capture* of the Jew (and exclusion of the non-Jew), which is what this paper is all about, seems less akin to religious than to Mafia membership, where it is understood there is no leaving it. To the "racial" argument, viz., that one can't change one's race, I would offer, besides the multicolored composition of the group worldwide, that such a high percentage of interbreeding gives that dubious thesis the lie.

Elliott Oring (1984) develops the thesis that Freud struggled over the "Jewish question" personally, his father having become Reform and practically areligious, before reaffirming his own affiliation.

No doubt one of the central issues in his conflict was the powerful incentive not to betray his father, which became intensely compounded when Jakob's belief was at variance with that of *his* historical father*s*. This might help account for the apparent retreat in Sigmund's own growing irreligiosity, and the paradoxical phenomenon in Jewish culture at large of the reversion to greater orthodoxy intergenerationally rather than a progressive attenuation over time.

Oring points out that many prominent middle-European 19th century Jews had a similar history, such as Theodore Herzl and Karl Marx: the former was an assimilationist before becoming a Zionist, the latter was baptized. Of course the Reform Judaism movement itself arose in the middle of that century in Germany.

Nicholas Horowitz speculates that cultural Darwinism has been at work in this group, with the living conditions so onerous that the strongest have survived by escaping, leaving within the accumulation of the *un*-fittest to inbreed. This *un*-adaptedness of the isolated remainder group inexorably has evolutionary consequences when the environment changes: witness, for

Let My People Go!: An Essay On Jewish Atavism And Theocracy.

one, the near extinction of the European breeding group and its gene pool in the Holocaust. Darwin's law could be paraphrased as *"Adapt or Die!"*

The prevalence of conversion may illuminate the matter further. Late-age conversion *out* of Judaism (often to Catholicism) seems to be a regular feature of the intellectuals, such as Gustav Mahler, the composer, Gregory Zilboorg, the psychoanalyst, and Mortimer Adler, the academic philosopher, in contrast to *in*-conversion in late age which is so rare as to be newsworthy. The difference is reminiscent of the hundreds of thousands or millions of Jews attempting to escape Soviet Russia, the bare handful in the other direction (yet another example of contemporary imprisonment of Jews and their victimology). The intriguing question is whether the out-converting intellectuals *also* felt they were freeing themselves from bondage, reflecting the *religion* as the oppressor.

When will the *multitude* of Jews cry, "Enough, already! We are tired of this role!"? I am aware of the motto "Never again!" of the Jewish Defense League and entirely sympathetic with their aims as is evident here. We both are too easily marginalized and discounted by the polite Jewish society, however. The necessity to have to fight for one's self is still experienced as not quite ego-syntonic, though embarrassedly prideful even when practiced by Israel. This is another manifestation of the persistent mentality of the oppressed in the character of the Jew, I believe: "Don't make trouble!" . You know the story: two Jews were facing the firing squad; one spat in the officer's face, the other advised prudence.

Extrapolating from my patient series, it could be that many Jews had a conflict as children over their desire to identify with their families versus a native revulsion to that to which they are exposed in their culture, particularly the experience of being held prisoner *by* their religion. Instant branding by their ritualistic traditions, however, and already established reciprocal social hatred toward them and by them guarantees the "prejudice" which keeps the young from straying. This is the external snare.

Let My People Go!: An Essay On Jewish Atavism And Theocracy.

Internally, the rabbis, like the priest class of many religions, or the "high priests" of any institution, social club or professional organization, exercise their political power to capture their constituencies by first condemning them with the voice of ultimate authority to be *out*, (and here the minority and condemned status of the Jews admirably serves this purpose and is thereby worth preserving), then offering protection or salvation by inviting them *in*. Priests who double as theocrats have twice the influence, authority, threat, and power to capture their flock and retain them than either spiritual counselors or secular governors alone...and are understandably loath to relinquish it. *It was therefore in the interest of the ancient rabbinate to preserve the beleaguered status quo of their constituencies vis-a-vis the greater society, which preserved their own power and even existence.*

Except, interestingly, in recent years over 50% of American Jews intermarry, genetically, when they get the chance to start their own families, voting thereby "with their feet" (not to mention the significant proportion who *never* marry, being unable to successfully resolve their conflict). However, many do not religiously, for they choose their partners exogamously and then convert them as a guilty retreat from the *apostasy* of the intermarriage. But the tendency to *out*-marry seems to be a general ethnic tendency in contemporary America, no doubt in part due to the social mixing and tradition of independence which exist here (Americans are no more obedient to Papal authority than Mosaic).

So the intermarriage phenomenon paradoxically may prove to have exactly the opposite effect than it seems to, actually serving to *conserve* the Jewish ethnic identity in the face of general societal diffusion, as well as providing the genetic diversity essential to the preservation of the breeding group. Here can be seen a striking example of the divergence between the instinctive, adaptive, essentially self-preserving impulse of the socialized and secularized Westernized Jew versus the de-evolutionary and thus self-defeating, religiously "pure" atavistic forces which look backward for preservation of the culture.

Let My People Go!: An Essay On Jewish Atavism And Theocracy.

Of pertinence to the thesis of this essay is one of the chief dynamic psychological motivations for intermarriage: for the Jewish partner, seeking acceptable *freedom and independence* from his nexus, for the Protestant partner, seeking acceptable *integration and dependence* into his nexus.

They wear their shame, the opposite of self-esteem, on their heads since the Spanish Inquisition, just as they were forced to wear the Star of David in Nazi Germany, and now memorialize their indignity in the death camps (which, like the historical oppression, "must not be forgotten!").

The original marking is, of course, the circumcision. The greater society always has and always will attack and try to destroy that which is different, especially if additionally it represents the worst in itself projected, which unfortunately is the scapegoat role assigned to and accepted by the classic Jew. The Christian has tried to proselytize, induce, and even force the Jew to believe, to redeem and save him as is *their* belief, but is his usefulness as a bogeyman self-limiting of these efforts?

It could be said that what the Egyptians and successor slave-masters projected into their Jewish subjects, the Jews have re-projected back into their historical and contemporary anti-Semites, both inciting revulsion at unacceptable psychic contents, and neither being faithful perceptions of the other group or themselves. Thus the difficulty with the projective solution to internal conflict is that it not only fails to resolve the problem but compounds the felony, rendering internal threats into external enemies which still need to be defended against, and leaving the subject group no better able to recognize and amend itself.

The central denigrated self-image is denied and glorified into the idea of being God's chosen people (with an ironic twist to the meaning of "chosen"), which air of superiority itself represents the return of the repressed, the ugliness of the boast.

This provocation of attack by bragging is related to their attempt to induce envy toward themselves by ostentatious behavior, intended to accomplish the denial and projection of their own envy toward the greater

Let My People Go!: An Essay On Jewish Atavism And Theocracy.

society. However, as with all projections the matter doesn't't end there, for the Jew is then compelled to defend himself from the (provoked) attacks by invoking the protective spirit, kayn aynhoreh, which shields him from the evil eye of envy.

The invention of their God as the one and only, Monotheism, in turn gave them the status of His one and only people, an undoubted source of the arrogance of primogeniture, reflected not only in this tribal motto but the claims of first or spiritual ownership of the Holy Land in the face of not being the first historical occupants. Not only is this one of the sources of the contemporary shoving match taking place there, but can be seen on the larger canvas to have contributed to the re-introduction of religious self-righteousness, intolerance, and provocation of competition in general, as other religions naturally took their Gods as first, also, while condemning Jews for their chutzpah.

The "First"s found ubiquitously chiseled over American Christian churches and financial institutions was a claim originally asserted by the Jews, now taken over and asserted by their competitors as an integral part of the notion of monotheism. Religious tolerance would be a respectful acceptance of others having their own gods, but of course that reintroduces pan-theism. What a clever maneuver: I have discovered (invented) the most important thing in all existence, there is only one of them, and I have it, not you!

The combinative "Judeo-Christian" is a term undoubtedly invented by Christians, respectfully acknowledging their historical and moral patrimony from the Jews. The Jews, on the other hand, are not equally comfortable about acknowledging their rival progeny, for "They shall have no other Gods before" them. This lack of reciprocity is also reflected in the Christians including portions of the Jewish Bible in their own, but not vice versa.

To the argument that this is only "natural", consider the relations between the revolutionary child America and its rebuffed parent England:

within only a relatively few years, the interchange of cultural characteristics between the two demonstrated a cross-identification which "credited" both. The Jews, on the other hand, seem to play the role of the spoiled spoilers toward their rivals, discrediting and adamantly refusing to recognize their legitimacy (echoes of the Holy Land today?). This is the pathognomonic sign of envy at work.

Mer. of Ven., IV,i,123, Gratiano: "...but on thy soul, harsh Jew,...no metal can...bear half the keenness of thy sharp envy."

The "badness" also returns as the bad public image they "suffer" (and take pains to cultivate). This to protect their central fear of assimilation, or loss of the distinction of their difference, which represents on the one hand a denial of the wish for the exact opposite, and on the other, marks the fixation of the individual and group psychological development at the narcissistic level, preventing further maturation, individuation, and identification with the rest of humanity.

This lack of individuation renders the cultural group un-democratic and socialistic, and stifles the young in their "search for themselves".

Mer. of Ven., I,iii,34, Shylock: "Yes, to smell pork; to eat of the habitation which your prophet the Nazarite conjured the devil into. I will buy with you, sell with you, talk with you, walk with you...but I will not eat with you, drink with you, nor pray with you."

The resistance to "taking in" from the surrounding society is typical of paranoid/narcissistic operations, not as much to protect against overt poisoning as the more subtle fear of "falling under the influence" and becoming just like everyone else.

This strenuously maintained difference and opposition to the greater society is manifested by idiosyncratic dress and language, social custom, diet, and ancient time system with its unique calendar, clock, and even inverted day/night cycle. "Jewish time" is known in the language. Jews

Let My People Go!: An Essay On Jewish Atavism And Theocracy.

greet strangers with the equivalent of a fraternity password, inquiring discreetly whether the newcomer is "M.O.T.?" ("Member Of the Tribe?") to be accepted unquestioningly or treated formally (shunned). No wonder Jews are the visitors in all the societies on earth, without national loyalty, and in the perfect position to both exploit that society which exploited them and be mistrusted by it.

A common example of this tribal provincialism is the not infrequent practice of educated Jews seeking out the familiar synagogue in a strange land, in preference to becoming acquainted with the repositories of Western Civilization such as the Parthenon, Vatican, Louvre, and Westminster. These are the same people who would scoff at the parochialism of visiting a familiar McDonald's eatery in Moscow, e.g.

It will be interesting to see whether the establishment of their own homeland will change how Jews see themselves, individually and as a group, vis-à-vis the greater society. However, as of a half-century later, Jews all over the world on Passover and elsetimes still anachronistically recite the prayers to be freed from bondage and to return to Jerusalem someday! Is this not convincing vestigial evidence of the contemporary survival of an historic slave mentality?

To the argument that slave-like characteristics must be proven rather than inferred to be believable, is to turn the task of the psychoanalytic ethnologist upon its head. The time-tested doctrines of "Ontogeny recapitulates Phylogeny" (the principle that early stages in biologic evolution of species are repeated in the embryonic development of the contemporary individual), and "the Child is Father to the Man" in the psychological development of the individual, both of these doctrines dictate that the naive and unnatural idea that a cultural group can have undergone a period of slavery in its past without there being any residuum, that is the hypothesis, I would say phantasy, which requires proof rather than vice versa.

Besides, that phantasy is contradicted by the commonplace observation that the historical experience remains very much alive in the ritual of the religion, and in the minds and on the lips of all observing Jews. The real question is whether it remains alive in their character and their culture, the thesis of this paper; a sense of conviction about that will only come with a gradual assembling of heretofore buried (repressed) characteristics which in the aggregate will deliver a subjective sense of "rightness" ...what I have come to after a long and painful period of discovery, and which each reader will have to experience for himself.

Fledgling Israel could be thought of as a cultural laboratory, a new direction in adaptedness in part compelled by the evolutionary catastrophe which befell the Jews during WWII. Here we can see under our very eyes the adaptive (secular) forces arrayed against the atavistic (zealously theocratic) ones in a dynamic struggle for survival, the outcome of which is of course unknowable.

We can not doubt and hope that the future of the Jews is not in the past. (As Gertrude Stein might have put it, "When there is only what was, then no will be" will be.) Here also we can see the proud modern citizen-Jew taking his place amongst the family of nations, the momentous result referred to below. For the non-Israeli Jew, however, the pathway will have to be different, although the very existence of the Jewish state has, or could have depending on future events, profound effects on the psyches of all Jews everywhere. As outlined in Part VII, possibly the European Jews, true to their history, are expending their efforts in re-establishing the ancient Hebrew nation, while the American Jews, true to theirs, are in increasing numbers Declaring their Independence.

To visualize how the Jews see themselves and others see them, conduct the following experiment, if you will. Imagine Israel, in your memory or the imago in the popular press. Do you see a poster of a young smiling couple looking to the future with sleeves rolled up, he muscular, she with tidy bandana, in their orchard making the desert bloom; perhaps with a proud khakied sentry guarding the outpost? Or do you see the popular emblem of the State, not the flag nor the olive branch but the Wailing wall with a black-hatted and frock-coated, hirsute and hair-suited, zealot bobbing and rocking in onanistic reverie?

Let My People Go!: An Essay On Jewish Atavism And Theocracy.

II

What would we imagine to be the characteristics of the psychology of slaves, since obviously none of us have ever worked with them? First, we suppose they would feel marked, and that the marking would have been imposed from without, given, leaving them powerless to change it. That would render them feeling different, exceptional, picked out and picked on; separated from the rest of humankind, they would live segregated, clustered, and insular. Their perspective would be narrow, low, parochial, unworldly. They would feel inferior, inadequate, lacking in self-esteem, unworthy; then punished, guilty after the fact, perhaps responsible. (A kernel of truth might reside there, in that their underlying warm, open, and somewhat passive nature, as well as their defensive aggressive provocativeness, might have rendered them vulnerable to have been taken slave in the first place.)

They would feel ineligible to take their rightful place among the society of men and nations, being without citizenship; ineligible and unable both, dependent as they are on the larger society for their existence, even as slaves. They would be subservient but with a covert arrogance, born of their ability to survive the worst thrown at them and the sense of moral superiority over their brutish overlords, plus a hidden identification with them. The males likely would feel castrated, limited to the work no one else would do, the females compensatorily empowered: thus the sons would tend to be mother-identified. They would tend to remain regressed and childish, unable to walk upright amongst their fellow-men.

They would feel persecuted, and that out of (projected) envy. They might feel suspicious of attempts to assist them as having the aim to re-oppress them. They definitely would feel as the outsider, unable to identify with the dominant society, but able to observe and criticize it. Having found their identity in their slavehood, they would be naturally reluctant to relinquish it. That slave identity would be superordinate to any other, (e.g. human, gender, name, nationality), rendering them almost irrelevant. A mood of victimization and masochism would be as second nature, as would be an easy camaraderie with their fellows and mistrust of strangers. Along with an acute sensitivity to cruelty might coexist a surprising numbness to it when practiced between themselves.

They would experience chronic depression, and perhaps as one resultant, heightened sensitivity, reflectiveness, and creativity; a lively emotionality and colorfulness as well as an intellectual curiosity might substitute for external freedom. Another underlying mood might be apathy and a tendency to surrender; resignation might lead to a sense of humor, of the self-deprecating variety. There would be no notion of redemption, neither in this life nor any other, nor for their children; this might be manifested in a fatalistic, nihilistic, and disillusioned outlook. At the same time, they might also feel aggressive, stubbornly oppositional, rebellious, unaccepting of the norms and values of the dominating society, cynical, heretical, vengeful, overtly attacking or insidiously sabotaging.

When their circumstances improved, perhaps by liberation, the now ex-slave might struggle against tendencies to assuage his deprivations with indulgences, by way of self-comforting food, materialistic luxuries, and status symbols ("nigger-rich"); or oppositely, to retain his former restrictions.

Does any of this bear similarity to the group psychology we are examining, and reciprocally, does the existence of any of these characteristics in the group have any probative value in our thesis, that they derive from historical slavehood?

III

The author (1990) describes a certain sub-group of under-parented patients who responded to being abandoned by becoming fixated at the level of secondary narcissism and erecting their own unconscious phantasied father who, in his perfectionistic, unforgiving demandingness, imprisoned the subject in a pleasureless defeated existence, ameliorated only by a megalomanic phantasy, one aspect of which was the (delusional) idea that he was his own father to himself (cf. the lordly Lordless Jew).

Let My People Go!: An Essay On Jewish Atavism And Theocracy.

That is, not only did he feel himself to be a punished victim, but that he was the moral judge himself, his own god. There co-existed two diametrically-opposed identities: a thoroughly abased individual (the son) and a completely ennobled one (the father) in the same person, the whole constituting a self-sufficient system requiring no external objects. (Ernest Jones, in his beautiful paper on The God Complex, details at length the connection between narcissistic traits and the phantasy of being the Supreme Being.) This, then, could provide a possible basis of that character trait of the individual Jew of being both the master and the slave.

Another relevant observation of these patients is their unremitting destructive hostility to newly-arrived rivals, their siblings. The parallel with the ongoing struggle with their neighbors by Israel compels itself to mind.

To extend the analogy and speculation yet further, these unparented children had an earlier history of conflictful (narcissistic) overindulgence by their mothers which preceded conflicts with their father and eventual abandonment, which raises at least three intriguing ideas which cannot be pursued further here: 1) that the Jewish psyche may contain frozen paleological evidence of an historical period of plenty and abundance, a veritable "Garden of Eden", finding memorialization in their religious mythology and their self-appointed identity as "chosen"; 2) that this psychohistorical period of plenty succeeded by one of desertification may be repeated each generation in the apparent ethnic practice of indulging their children, the promise of which is never met by later reality, which consequently is experienced by the child as a desertion or abandonment by his "Gods" or fate, and a persisting attitude of disillusionment; 3) that the Jewish people seek to return to their historic "birthplace" to find their redemption, an area long since desertified but which they are determined to (re-) make bloom. (In passing, note the relationship between the noun and verb desert: the desert is that which has been deserted by [Mother] nature.) With these ideas, one is compelled to imagine a slave-mother seeking solace in an overly-invested infant, and a pubertal slave-boy being accorded the work obligations of a full-grown man, both images not at all discordant with the psychology and practices of the Jew.

Therapeutic contact with a live and present uncondemning surrogate father, the coming to grips with the unconscious sense of abandonment, rage, badness and compensatory omnipotence, offers the only possibility of change in these patients. The phenomenon serves as a paradigm of what we are discussing on a group level here, corresponding to the unconscious cultural attitudes already discussed plus a new one: the intriguing religious belief that the Jews are still awaiting their savior.

IV

Christianity has been postulated as a further development and evolution of Judaism, which remained fixated at an earlier stage. In our conception, too, the severe, punishing "Old Testament God" of the Jews could be viewed as an incorporation of the slave-master and/or the creation of a phantasied demanding God-father to replace the one who had abandoned and forsaken them into slavery.

The "Loving God" of the Christians, on the other hand, achieved the emancipation, the dignity, and even the nobility of man by the device of forgiving of his "original" sin or badness, and by being present. In this view, Christians are not practicing merely an alternative religion, but have achieved an emancipation of their formerly Jewish slave status. They have thrown off their internal bonds, their constructed and/or incorporated slave-master, and can rejoice "on high". A loving God has indeed been the savior of the Christians.

Here is a bit of internal evidence of Christ's actuality, and by inference, the therapeutic effect of a real versus an imagined father. An important distinction resides here: the Christian has a relationship with an external (and real, and human) God, to whom he is subordinate, and between them his religious leader, also a "servant of God", serves as an intermediary. He may have a touch of godliness in him to the extent that he is a devout subject, but he remains the subject. The God of the Jews and their rabbinical theocrats is, on the other hand, phantastic and personified in both the religious leader and the subjects themselves...they behave as though they think they are the God...lending an opposite quality of arrogance rather than humility.

Let My People Go!: An Essay On Jewish Atavism And Theocracy.

Moses brought down the law; his successors laid down the law. This self-appointed "mission" of law-giver or conscience of society is what confers a quality of provocative insufferability on Jews, stimulating guilt and counterattacks by the other members of society and by Jews themselves toward themselves.

To the extent the Christians have been absolved by shifting blame to the Jews and thereby instituting scapegoating, however, their emancipation has been at the expense of those left behind. Jesus took the sins of man upon himself to save them by self-sacrifice, but it was this necessity to sacrifice himself which is the underlying source of the blame of the Jews, not the political or temporal conditions of the crucifixion itself which is often the locus of the debate.

Interestingly, on the one hand the early Christian converts from Judaism were viewed as apostates, began their existence as slaves, and were persecuted unmercifully by the Romans as the Christian martyrs, but that experience did not become incorporated into their religion and become worn as a badge of their faith; i.e., the historical experience is not a necessary condition for the erection of a harsh god.

To be sure there exists a variety of masochism in the Christian character which can be every bit as virulent as in any other; however, its basis may be different, consisting in guilt over enjoying after their savior suffered to make that possible, or an identification with humble, willing and ennobling self-sacrifice, rather than imposed, vengeful and demeaning punishment.

On the other hand, there exist other "Old Testament"-fixated or atavistic sects, many with ascetic characteristics, such as Islamic fundamentalists, Christian Amish, Hindu fakirs and Buddhist monks, all physically and psychologically resembling classic Jews in their harsh mode of existence and confrontational opposition to 21st century society (other-worldliness). These, too, would be postulated as having been originally caused by the incorporation of a severe God-taskmaster, and/or the creation of a phantasied perfectionistic God-father to replace the one who had abandoned them and who had been abandoned in turn.

The contemporary prevalence of these fundamentalist sects and the dynamic conflict with their secular cultural opposite numbers, repeated in many societies and eras and notable currently would be a reactive oscillation to perceived excesses in the opposite direction, including the sense that the society and their God had both abandoned each other. Thus, the "return to fundamentals".

Joan Lachkar (1983) postulates in her dissertation the thesis that the mythology of the Arab Moslems reveals their psychology to be that of abandonment. But that is essentially not dissimilar to the Jews, at least latently, though covered with their manifest opposite claim. She also points out that the Arabs, among others, had a prior claim to the Holy Land.

Their religion without doubt was the preserver of the Jews as a society while in bondage and exile. It remains to be seen whether they can achieve the same spiritual emancipation as the Christians without leaving their faith now that they have been free for several millennia, by extrojecting their Pharaonic and successor Judaic theocratic overlords and their accompanying burden of psychic detritus, (which may involve acknowledging their sense of badness and seeking forgiveness, if only from themselves) and incorporating historical and contemporary Jewish (and universal) heroes ("gods") having land, dignity, and acceptance in the world's society.

What may be a case in point is the contemporary movement amongst American Negroes (the group which shares with Jews a history of enslavement, looking to others to rescue them, and castrated males within a matriarchal family; the group with which Jews feel spiritually akin) to redefine their own identity and restore their own dignity by discarding their inherited but originally adopted last names and Christian religion of their slavemasters (reflecting their hidden identification), and adopting of the Islamic religion and naming. One may anticipate that this will fail in its intended result, however, in that they have exchanged one slave-master for another, but it is an undeniable attempt at self-emancipation. The "Black Pride" effort to educate their own and others of their race's accomplishments and contributions to the greater society seems, on the other hand, a worthy effort to emulate.

V

In the sifting process which needs accompany contemplating these ideas, it would seem useful to distinguish between form and substance in the belief system which is Judaism. Substance, like much of the Talmud's accumulated wisdom about human nature, conduct, and morality is unchanging, precious, and to be studied and assimilated for the pursuit of the good life, along with the moral teachings of many other civilizations and authors, no single one possessing a monopoly on wisdom.

On the other hand, some of the ur-ancient time-dated rituals, beliefs and prayers, the forms of the religion may, in their irrelevancy to contemporary life, serve to undermine the very values they propose to conserve. For a reasonably healthy (modern American) individual who is not so inclined, for instance, some practices are repugnant merely because of their undeniable similarity to the symptomatic thoughts and rituals of Obsessive-Compulsive, Paranoid, Masochistic and Narcissistic illnesses. This personal reaction plus the realization of the gratuitous difficulties other Jews have made for his life can form the nucleus of the individual's own private Jewish anti-Semitism, undoubtedly more widely experienced than publicly acknowledged: and all without any necessary implication of sinister motives. However, the reaction-formation against these feelings is typical of the practicing Jew.

It has been postulated that religious and political movements often institutionalize the individual neurosis or psychosis of the founder, which finds fertile soil in the Zeitgeist and psyches of his followers.

For the children in particular, emphasizing positive accomplishments which can be admired rather than persecutions endured, which only reinforce a negative self-image, would seem to be especially cogent.

Let My People Go!: An Essay On Jewish Atavism And Theocracy.

Being taught Hebrew by the last remaining unemployed scholar-tutor in the community, often a bearded, spittle-flecked, urine-stained smelly elder, is not particularly admirable to a young child, either.

Likewise, it would seem to be helpful for Jewish organizations to lift their sights beyond parochial concerns to other groups and universal problems to demonstrate their underlying identification with others. Why have not the Jews, with all their resources and intellect, established a number of general universities like the Baptists?

To the extent that the religious group reflects a fixation at an early (secondary narcissistic) level of development, with the focus on the helplessness/grandiosity of its subjects in the sway of/unneedful of a severe (absent) lord, with a self-centered world-view, struggle against relations and identification with others, and the non-achievement of personhood, it could be said the problem is to continue the stalled development, or grow up! This would entail accepting: being like everyone else, and responsibility for the way they are, appear to others, and the consequences of their own actions (rather than being resigned to their underlying sense of powerlessness/satisfied with their granted perfection, both of which lead to injustice-collecting, and blaming and manipulating others to rectify their disadvantaged lives). This is why the grievances "must not be forgotten!".

To the argument that the 20th century enslavement and near extinction cannot be allowed to happen again, I would offer that the best protection would be the overcoming of shame and re-establishment of authentic Jewish pride, which the celebration of the memories of suffering directly undermines; the relinquishment of their childish passivity for adult responsibility for themselves in Jewish self-defense; and the confronting of the unsettling proposition that Jews as a cultural group preoccupied with its past have a self-perpetuating master/slave mentality and society.

Shame is the natural reaction to the loss of bodily or emotional control, originating in the experience of excretory incontinence and arising from the failure to reach expected levels of behavior in one's own ideal. It constitutes

Let My People Go!: An Essay On Jewish Atavism And Theocracy.

a powerful incentive to develop self-control or continence, which, along with the acquisition of skills leads to its opposite, pride. Guilt, on the other hand, is a tension between the group's incorporated moral conscience and oneself which compels one to punish oneself or "do right", particularly in one's treatment of others.

In our contemporary politically indulgent American culture, what used to be or should be one group's shame (e.g. not learning the language or earning a living) is externalized into another group's blame and attendant guilt, with predictable results: the nominated responsible society futilely attempts to rid itself of guilt while the errant group even magnifies its behavior. Thus we are left with a vicious cycle of a shameless and guilt-ridden society. What has been our shame and guilt must be owned up to, to be rectified; what is others' is theirs to do the same.

To the extent that the religion represents the symbolic castration of the men, with the compensatory empowerment of the women (the prototypical "Jewish mother"), the problem is to recover that male wholeness which has been lost in order to restore his integrity, his Jewish potency (as contrasted with his omnipotency/impotency). There is a body of belief (based on exploration of mens' unconscious) that ceremonial circumcision plays a significant but not exclusive role in the problem, which has been losing favor even as a hygienic measure world-wide in recent decades. Judaism seems much more congenial to women than to men, and to womens' work (priests and doctors, viz. men with skirts).

William Sheldon (1944), the physical anthropologist, in a personal communication was struck by the maleness of the Jewish females and vice versa in his various psychological and anthropometric indices, peculiar to this group alone. Besides this point of gender diffusion, his work should chasten us not to over-psychologize the issue of character traits in general, for there may well be an inherited element in this and other breeding group's characteristics: in fact, lacking evidence to the contrary, we might assume there is.

Let My People Go!: An Essay On Jewish Atavism And Theocracy.

Cf. the South American psychoanalytic literature regarding the growing abandonment of male circumcision. Indirectly but with intriguing inference, Samuel Lipton (1962) observes that for at least 2,500 years man has practiced the mutilative surgery tonsillectomy, in the recent century the most prevalent surgical procedure (after circumcision), without a sound basis in theory and having no lasting medical utility, which leads him to conclude that it is merely a crypto-ritual with predominantly psychological significance.

In this schema, then, the combination of the rituals of neonatal circumcision and pubertal bar Mitzvah both reflect, reinforce, and perpetuate the dual problem of the Jews' self-conception, viz., that of the captive and innocently-injured (martyred), and pretentiously and presumptuously superior (grandiose), creditor of special treatment. What this amounts to is the feminization of the male.

Circumcision involves relinquishing a symbolic portion of masculinity, an effect which has been amply elaborated in the psychoanalytic literature. Likewise, studying for and taking the bar Mitzvah ceremony involves again relinquishing a portion of masculinity, in that the novice is precluded from "joining other boys" in their afterschool activities (sports, etc.), a highly symbolic and actual deprivation experienced by the boy as such, who is made to comply instead with the ideal of being a "good boy", (not dissimilar in intent if not timing from the Catholic practice of training their altar and choir boys), and with similar and now compounded feminizing effect.

The assertion that "today I am a man", in addition to being pretentious absurd, is a thin denial of the exact opposite. Unlike the initiation rites of passage in primitive tribes where the boys eschew the women and their incorporated qualities and join the men, the Jewish ceremony signals the joining of the feminized, impotent, scholarly half-men (described by William Sheldon many years ago, and re-discovered by every Jewish male in psychoanalysis).

Thus is generated anew within each individual the narcissistic claim, which in turn requires the application of religious mythology and further ritual by the theological authorities, thereby insuring their survival also, the whole constituting a self-perpetuating vicious cycle. What the Canaanites (vide infra) addressed with the label of the "disease of Judaism", we would then agree resembles a socially-induced individual and group neurosis or character disorder, not unknown in other human societies and times.

VI

Published or discovered after completion of this paper are ten apropos publications, which typify the kind of library research remaining to flesh out this thesis:

1) Stanley Rothman (1978) quotes Ferdinand Lassalle (1862) corresponding with Karl Marx about their mutual views of Jews: "I see in them nothing but the degenerate sons of a great but long past epoch. As a result of centuries of servitude these people have taken on the characteristics of slaves...".

Also of interest to us is his observation that Jews constituted the overwhelming majority in the radical revolutionary movements in Russia and Cuba, the American Communist Party, and the American counter-culture movement of the 60's. We would note that such an undermining of the institutions of the greater society obviously provokes the antipathy and counter-attacks of that society, thereby creating the very oppression suffered. We would additionally note that the Bolsheviks, mostly Jews, became the oppressors in the new society after rebelling against the oppression in the old; this fact may be one of the major sources of the resurgent anti-Semitism amongst the newly liberated masses.

2) Howard Stein (1978) states, "My clinical judgment, psycho-historically derived, is that Jews have unconscious complicity in their history. Jews have been, and remain, active victims (not passive casualties) of their group-fantasy whose core is martyrdom (...victimology)."

3) Jay Gonen (1975) traces the original Hebrew nation through the successor Jewish religion to the current Zionist Israeli nation, a secular nationalistic movement which is both forward-looking and attempting the

recapture of the glory of the old Kingdom, but also to elide the intervening Jewish theocracy (which of course is struggling to preserve itself). He quotes the modern Canaanite movement which distinguishes between the original Hebrew nation and its successor, the Jewish religion, which it labels unabashedly as a disease.

Julius Wellhausen (1957), Gonen continues, distinguished between the pre-exilic Israel and post-exilic Judaism," which was the result of a rise of a theocracy...and the metamorphosis of a great idea into an institution. The new Judaism 'left no free scope for the individual'. This deadening cultus was the means employed to preserve 'a religious community even after all bonds of nationality had fallen away'. Oswald Spengler developed his own notions concerning the enfeeblement of the Jewish people ever since the Babylonian Exile".

Gonen further says, "The origins of the negative ego-ideal were clearly to be found in the shameful Galut (Exile), with its related dispersion, persecutions, expulsions, pogroms, homelessness, and helplessness." Discussing Whitman's and Kaplan's (1968) treatment of the concept of negative identity, he says, "...(the Jew) may perceive himself as a jerk, slob, klutz, schnorrer, sad sack or schlemiehl."

He also wrote of the dangers of the "Masada Complex" which has been warned about by Menahem Begin among many others: the idea There is no tomorrow! Begin challenged, "Never another Masada", and advocated the achievement of honor through victory, life, and freedom rather than by an honorable death.

In a brief biographical note, Gonen reveals he is a native-born Sabra who identifies himself as a non-Jewish Hebrew!

4) The 1990 National Jewish Population Survey (Conducted by Barry A. Kosmin et al, reported in the Los Angeles Times of August 6, 1991 by Gary Libman) found Orthodox Jews to constitute less than 7% of the American religious group (and Hasidim a tiny percentage of that)

belying their apparent number ostentatiously parading in the community and media, but when combined with those self-identified as Conservative, comprise almost half of the American group, the other half representing Reform and miscellaneous; this is a ratio similar to the religious/secular political grouping in Israel.

The survey also uncovered some "sobering" statistics (we would say surprising only to hard-shelled patriarchs who assumed their constituents were marching lock-step behind them): that in the intermarried families 72% of the children are raised without a Jewish education, and over 90% of them out-marry! But, 60% of intermarried couples responded that being Jewish was important to them, in spite of not educating their children in the religion...suggesting to us that indeed the intermarriage may be preserving the breeding group and the ethnic identity but not the religion.

Sociologist Bruce Phillips of Hebrew Union College, quoted in the same article, noted that prior waves of Jewish immigration to America, Sephardics in Colonial times and German Jews in the 1840's, disappeared into the general population by the fourth generation, which he opines is happening now with the last wave of Russian immigration of the 1880-1900's.

5) Manfred Weidhorn (1992) has contributed a beautifully-written essay on the sources of anti-Semitism in Jews themselves, which sources he exhorts Jews to confront before trying to assign the ("lion's share "of the) blame to "Christendom".

6) Albert Lindemann (1992) posits one important source of anti-Semitism in the actual "rising of the Jews" demographically, socio-economically and politically with the relaxation of restrictive laws in various European countries, and their seeming over-running of the host society. This is reflected in his citation of a dedicated anti-Semite Edouard Drumont (1844-1917), author of La France juive (Jewish France), "...the dream of the Semite...his obsession, has always been to reduce the Aryan to servitude." We, of course, detect an equally real and deeper dimension to this observation.

Let My People Go!: An Essay On Jewish Atavism And Theocracy.

The author underscores the reality of Jewish aggressive business and political practices as also leading to the society's counter-reaction, a point commonly denied in discussions of this subject but very much in the awareness of critics of Jews. Altogether, in many contexts, he emphasizes the reality of the complaints against the Jews, whether distorted, exaggerated, or misplaced. With this observation we agree, and would only add that the surface manifestations which are experienced as provocative only mirror deeper intentions (and are correctly read by the greater society and reacted to). Here is a link to Stein's observation that Jews are not merely passive victims but active shapers of their own victimology.

Lindemann also cites Jewish poet Heinrich Heine's acerbic observation, "'Those who would say that Judaism is a religion would say that being a hunchback is a religion. 'For him, Judaism was not a religion but a 'misfortune'".

7) Rabbi Ephraim Buchwald in the Los Angeles Times of April 28, 1992, claims that the morbid preoccupation with the Holocaust is "killing off" a whole generation of young Jews who see nothing in the religion but "the spectre of endless victimization and suffering". "We must make certain that young Jews who enter these (Holocaust) centers encounter a message that will inspire them to live as Jews:...positivism and joy."

"We've reached the absurd point where the only feature of Judaism with which our young Jews identify is that of the Jew as victim. Is there no joy...balm...in Jewish life? Unless we 'choose life', we are probably witnessing the last generation of Jewish life in America as we know it...the'silent Holocaust 'will have done its job, and Hitler will have emerged victorious."

8) Daniel Williams, in a piece entitled, "A Kinder, Gentler Zionism for Israel?", Los Angeles Times, August 4, 1992, reprises the cultural/political situation in Israel following the accession of the Labor party and Yitzhak Rabin to power in the recent elections, neatly highlighting many of the issues in this essay.

Let My People Go!: An Essay On Jewish Atavism And Theocracy.

He capsulizes, "The nationalist movement known as Zionism...founding father Theodore Herzl...who ironically believed that Jews should assimilate into Western secular culture (via) a homeland in Palestine. The nature of that homeland and its relation to the rest of the world has been a matter of ideological conflict ever since. One side strives for a country like any other, while the other side believes Israel must stress its uniqueness (emphasis added)."

"To Labor...Israel is meant to engender normalcy for a people long burdened by persecution; in Israel, Jews for the first time are meant to feel at ease with the world at large. The centuries-old 'Jewish Question' would be resolved by making Israel a state like others in the liberal, modern Western mold that Jews throughout history helped to construct. Within this stream of Zionism runs a strong...disregard for tradition: the whole late 19th century idea of leaving Europe's Jewish ghettos to return to the ancestral homeland in Palestine was, in part, a revolt against religious-centered Judaism (emphasis added). These Zionists were bent on creating a New Jewish Man, an identity nourished by the land, by work and security."

"To (the religious) others, this brand of Zionism...smacks of trying 'to pass' for non-Jew...and to heck with what outsiders think."

"Rabin...in his inaugural speech... 'It is our duty to ourselves and our children to see the new world as it is now, to discern its dangers, explore its prospects and do everything possible so that the State of Israel will fit into this world whose face is changing. No longer are we necessarily "A people that dwells alone" and no longer is it true that "The whole world is against us". We must overcome the sense of isolation that has held us in its thrall for almost half a century [?? How about 2 millenia? (Ed.)]...join the international movement toward peace.'"

"Aloni (the new Education minister) speaks approvingly of the need to bring outside influences into the life of Israel. By (naming) Aloni, Rabin was (asserting) an outward-looking Jewishness (emphasis added). "The article closes with the concluding remarks of Rabin: "The answer is within us; the answer is ourselves.". [To which we say, "Amen!".(Ed.)]

9) D'Ambola reminds us of the psychodynamic defense of displacement backwards in time, the preoccupation with historical grievances thus protecting against recognition of and dealing with contemporary ones.

10) Rabbi Hecht reviews the movie "Schindler's List", questioning the value of lionizing the "swindler" Schindler, and echoing the by-now familiar theme of how Holocaust museums and films serve to dis-incentivize young Jews from embracing their religion, linked as it is to victimization. "What we should be doing is teaching the richness and everlasting greatness of our noble religion and not the negative experiences."

VII

To attempt an integrating psychohistorical reconstruction:

The Hebrew tribes enjoy a period of prosperity and plenty.

The nation is defeated in war (?possibly as a consequence of that abundance) and the populace forced into slavery and then exile.

The polarity of the sense of identity is changed from positive to negative, with the incorporation of virulent self-hatred necessitating modification by psychic defense.

The conversion of victor into vanquished is rationalized as due to the abandonment by their formerly protective God, which idea is later reinforced by their years of wandering in exile, both states necessitating becoming physically, psychologically, and spiritually self-sufficient.

The felt loss of their prior God is substituted for by a created God of their own making, tending to be perfectionistic and harsh. The Jewish religion forms.

Let My People Go!: An Essay On Jewish Atavism And Theocracy.

The internalization of their own God and identification with His authority renders the Jews regressed from the former state of relations with others to one of self-containment or narcissism.

The regressive instinctual defusion yields large amounts of free aggressive drive energy, rendering the group unusually combative, both in its internal relations within itself and externally with others.

This released level of aggressivity is in addition to the pre-existing pre-capture base level in the breeding group, and will be further magnified by any defensive operations particularly directed at expected (projected and provoked) aggression from the outside.

The form of the aggressive discharges, at least through much of history, were typically passively expressed, indirect and covert to guard against retaliation, but have again emerged in rather direct form in Israel. The Sabras are fighters; were the ancient Hebrews?

The grandiosity thus effected is wrapped around a debased, self-enraged and thus depressed core.

The original self-esteem of the Hebrew nation, holding its own in the society of tribes and nations, has now given way to the false (delusional) pride of the religious culture of being chosen and its accompanying convictions of differentness and superiority (replacing the opposite humiliating perceptions, rendering the paradoxical picture of the "proud" slave).

Since they have already achieved worldly perfection, there is no felt need to examine themselves or their state of affairs, discounting outside criticism as products of hatred or envy of their superior status.

By the same token, this self-satisfaction blinds them to the virtues, values, and accomplishments of the greater society, rendering it anti-heroic and not to be emulated or joined.

Let My People Go!: An Essay On Jewish Atavism And Theocracy.

Having lost its nation, the group's only coherent force is its particularity, its ways, its culture, its religion, its situation of being embattled.

That is, the group turns its attention from outwards, from the world at large and its own role in it, to itself, superficially aggrandizing but more deeply depriving itself from the supplies, support, and rewards to be had there.

The initial identification with the aggressor Pharaohs and the later incorporation of the group's own (rabbinical) authority, plus the free aggression released by the regressed state, all work to render the group internally conflict-ridden and oppressed, matching the rejection originally imposed from without, now internally generated and thus mastered and under its own control (as in the case of adopting the yarmulke after its use was imposed during the Spanish Inquisition).

The religious leaders become also secular leaders or theocrats, again in the service of self (group) preservation, multiplying the power of the religion and its priests over its constituency.

The group and individual identity contains components of both master and slave, rendering the paradoxical picture of the self-sufficient arrogant captive(/captor).

The defeat and enslavement by the outside society, the negativity consequent to the sense of identity, plus the punitiveness felt in the interior from the combination of the incorporated taskmasters, the self-generated and -directed hostility, and the actual deprivation of societal companionship, all make for an insufferable climate of persecution, which has to be rationalized (from others' envy of their superiority), defended against (coherent embattlement), and re-projected (as coming from the exterior).

In addition, the intolerable persecution is reversed in direction from Jew to Gentile in the role of social conscience or critic.

Let My People Go!: An Essay On Jewish Atavism And Theocracy.

The whole recreates and preserves the climate of slavery, "edified" to include a noble cause and purpose. The Jews preempt and arrogate to themselves the role of law-givers and preservers of truth and virtue, thus the saviors of the greater society, winning few adherents in the process but instead succeeding in aggravating the original external oppression into a vicious cycle of martyrdom.

The total effect is a developmental fixation, with no growth over time, adaptation to changing circumstance, nor influence from the outside, and a preoccupation within the group with its own situation, history, and past, i.e., with itself.

This "inwardness" is correctly perceived by the outside society as hostile to it, and is thus provocative of reactions of counter-aggression. (Unlike the separateness of the Amish, e.g., who keep to themselves, the Jews insist on living in the greater society but never becoming part of it.)

The chief anxiety of this fixated developmental level is that of annihilation, stemming from the fusion anxiety of further regression with loss of self, and from the opposite progressive threat of attention to the outside, which also threatens the loss of self.

This internal and intrinsic psychological state of affairs is mirrored, not caused, in external reality via the situational fear of annihilation reflected in the Holocaust, the concern about Israel's security, and the fear of assimilation; and by the constant (paranoid) expectation of being wiped out.

One corollary is the felt need to capture and insure the retention of attention from the outside, for the flagging of it or its disappearance could also signal the dreaded annihilation. The group's problems become perpetual and everyone's.

External beings and cultures are not perceived as such in their own right, but as adjuncts to the centrality of the self, and as such, to be ignored or used as the desire demands.

Let My People Go!: An Essay On Jewish Atavism And Theocracy.

The chief modality of relating to external objects is through aggressive action on them, one variety of which is manipulation, the acting upon the responsive object to make it react in the desired direction.

The chief means of manipulation is through provocation, which can include arousing attention, guilt, counter-aggression, or desire (seduction).

The Jewish society reaches a point of relative stability in its coherence, isolation from the greater society, and structure of psychic defenses, relatively resistant to change and enduring over time, "preserving" the cultural group during its trials.

It becomes selected; persecuted, embattled, and victimized; innocent, virtuous, satisfied; critical, accusatory, and undermining: society's sacrificed saviors (martyrs) and trouble-makers (the Jewish Problem).

The isolated populace becomes highly but randomly inbred, rendering an abnormally large proportion of both gifted (thoroughbreds) and also defective or maladapted individuals, the breeding group lacking the refreshment and genetic balance of "hybrid vigor".

External societal as well as internal pressure builds over time for the better adapted to leave the group to the less well-adapted, further degrading the quality of the inbred group.

Forced conversion as well as spontaneous assimilation and emigration play a role in the continuing dispersal of the coherent cultural group, as distinguished from the dispersal of the whole group from its homeland known as The Diaspora.

In increasing numbers contemporary American as well as Israeli Zionist Jews become secularized.

The by-now coherently organized and self-contained Jewish society is able to live only in enclaves within the larger society, fixated at and repeating the

Let My People Go!: An Essay On Jewish Atavism And Theocracy.

experiences of isolation and rejection, and reinforcing the dynamic defenses which the rabbinate, the religion, and the psychology of the masses fashioned originally.

However, the Jewish "solution" to its problem of slavery, exile and dispersal, i.e., the construction of theocratic enclaves within the greater society, make a "Jewish problem" for that society by virtue of the Jews' isolation from, criticism and rejection of it, the society's perception of its own subversion, exploitation, and inability to make peace with its critics. In addition, the Jews' separateness, "superiority", and non-belief make them a convenient scapegoat for continuing religious persecution.

The Christian "solution" to the "Jewish problem" is vigorously defended against by the Jews whilst both secretly admired in the prophecy of awaiting their very own savior (as though Christ was not their own), as well as essentially adopting that role as a group, a group which claimed to have special access to God.

In fact, the claim has psychological truth, in the fact that the God is incorporated within the group and individual structure, thereby offering special access, indeed. This is but one aspect of the narcissistic fusion with the omnipotent object.

It could be said that the Jews, far from disowning Jesus as their own and denying his divinity, have instead unwittingly identified with his role, adapting it to their own religious group, feeling themselves to be the ultimate saviors of mankind, purveyors of the truth, and representatives of the deity. They are thus latent competitors of Christianity, not merely forbears or deniers of it.

The Nazi "solution" to the "Jewish problem" (consisting of a convenient scapegoat population of talented competitors to their hegemony, a nonproductive peasantry, and feared dilution of their genetic ambitions) was the attempted destruction of the breeding material, the aptly-named genocide.

Let My People Go!: An Essay On Jewish Atavism And Theocracy.

The Zionist "solution" of re-establishing the Hebrew nation was an understandable attempt to recapture the ancient glory of the tribe, to undo the intervening group "failures", and to preserve its genetic identity.

It failed to deal, however, with the interim establishment of the Jewish religion with its own entrenched theocracy and constituency (against which the infant nation is struggling mightily still, only slightly less so than with its external neighbors),...

...and with the American invention of individual liberty, which in sharply increasing numbers had Western Jews experiencing the whole problem as an irrelevancy ("Who needs it?").

Perhaps the apparent American "solution" of intermarriage to assimilate into and identify with the greater society and refresh the gene pool, whilst simultaneously preserving those aspects of Jewish culture felt to be valuable but eschewing those aspects of Jewish religion felt to be oppressive, is showing the way to the future adaptation and preservation of the Jewish culture.

To the extent that this social development is predicated on an outward turning to the greater society, a perception of the positive value of that society, a retention of valued aspects of their own heritage but a discarding of non-valued identifications, and a strong desire to be liberated from historic limitations, the modern Jewish movement into the 21st century can be said to be the product of psychological maturation, which augurs well for the future of Jews, not necessarily of the Jewish religion as constituted.

In their apparent repudiation of the religion, the Zionist and American Jews both seem to have reached a consensus in their search for freedom from oppression. The religion may have been apprehended thus indirectly to be the reservoir and transmitter of the slave mentality in the culture.

One can only speculate on the historical and social forces which have assisted this maturing and liberating process in the Jewish culture:

Let My People Go!: An Essay On Jewish Atavism And Theocracy.

One thinks of actual threats to continued existence, the devastation of the Holocaust and the continuing drain of assimilation,

As well as the new social order which is America, experienced by many over its recent history and now viewed by all via television.

It is hard to imagine the witnessing of identified-as-Jewish leaders and fighters playing a respected role on the world stage as not having had its influence, also.

VIII

To afford the reader perspective on the perspective of the author, my personal history is that of a first-generation American raised by immigrant parents, together two of fifteen siblings plus four parents from Eastern Europe who settled in the American Middle-west (in the same community, it might be noted, as Golda Meir). They were nominal Jews, observing only the High Holidays in temple, participating in a Gentile culture with predominantly Jewish friends and their tightly-knit extended family. Both were of Orthodox stock but determined to raise their two children in the Reform Temple, if any, and to become Americanized (e.g. my father was a proud Navy veteran of WWI and active member of the American Legion). My father (Rumanian) and sister (Rumanian and Polish) were blue-eyed blondes in their youth, myself blue-eyed and brunette.

I attended Sunday School in my adolescence only (studying Latin and German in public school, not Hebrew in private) and was confirmed at 16 chiefly because of my mother's alarm that all my friends were Gentile. Consequently I met young Reform Jews as friends, but never identified with their religious affiliation; I had only minimal contact with Orthodox ones. This lack of identification with either the minority or the majority society left me doubly un-culture-bound, though painfully isolated.

The heavily German society was strongly pro-Hitler before the war, but my personal exposure to anti-Semitism in a white suburb was only to the covert

Let My People Go!: An Essay On Jewish Atavism And Theocracy.

and polite variety. Traveling East in the military/college, I became aware of the huge metropolitan Jewish population collected there and of the heavy-duty anti-Semitic discrimination to match, being the only or token Jew in my group to obtain ready acceptance into medical school.

In my adult life, I have experienced the three major (Western) religions in my close relationships and have intermarried, as have almost all of my cousins on my father's side of the family, some of whom have even out-converted, and have determined to carry on and enhance the valued tradition of my father and his father, which is to minimize any religious indoctrination of my children.

I am a classical (or Orthodox if you will) psychoanalyst by training who in four decades of practice has evolved my own individual technique and a special interest in characterology, a derivative of narcissism, and has currently in preparation papers on WASPS, Catholics, unparented children, aggression, and aspects of the American society and character.

In this practice Jews and Christian Scientists have been strikingly over-represented, and there is possibly a dynamic connection between these two groups. The Christian Scientists frequently gave the childhood history of having been spurned by mother when in pain, instructed to go off by themselves and "pray to God" for their relief. The Jews gave no such history, instead just proved to feel depressed in the course of their treatment, an inferential product of the unconscious rejection and abandonment they felt from their God, according to the thesis of this paper. Both groups of patients are "object-seeking", looking for someone to listen to them, understand (be in touch with) them, and accept them, rendering them readily amenable to the psychoanalytic milieu. For the Scientist group, this is in sharp contrast to the refractoriness of many other WASP sects to treatment.

REFERENCES

Buchwald, Rabbi Ephraim. "The Holocaust is Killing America's Jews", The Los Angeles Times, Op-Ed page, April 28, 1992.

D'Ambola, John, M.D. Personal Communication, 1992.

Freud, Sigmund, M.D. Moses and Monotheism. SE London: Hogarth Press, 1964.

Gay, Peter, Ph.D. A Godless Jew. Freud, Atheism, and the Making of Psychoanalysis. New Haven and London: Yale University Press, and Cincinnati: Hebrew Union College Press, 1987.

Gonen, Jay Y., Ph.D., A Psychohistory of Zionism. New York: Mason/Charter, 1975.

Hecht, Rabbi Eli, "When Will Jews Let It Rest?", The Los Angeles Times, Op-Ed page January 2, 1994.

Horowitz, Nicholas A., B.A. Personal Communication.

Horowitz, William S., M.D. The Bootstrapper: A Contemporary Characterology. (unpublished), 1990.

Johnson, Paul. A History of the Jews. New York: Harper and Row, 1988.

Jones, Ernest, M.D. "The God Complex (1913)", Essays in Applied Psychoanalysis. London: Hogarth Press, 1951, 2:244-265.

Kosmin, Barry A. Exploring and Understanding the Findings of the 1990 National Jewish Population Survey. A paper prepared for the Hollander Colloquium, the University of Judaism, Los Angeles, July 1991.

Lachkar, Joan, Ph.D. Dissertation: "The Arab-Israeli Conflict".

Libman, Gary. "At A Crossroads", The Los Angeles Times, August 6, 1991.

Lindemann, Albert S., Ph.D. The Jew Accused; Three Anti-Semitic Affairs (Dreyfus, Beilis, Frank) 1894-1915. Cambridge: Cambridge University Press, 1992.

Lipton, Samuel, M.D. "On the Psychology of Childhood Tonsillectomy", The Psychoanalytic Study of the Child, V. 17. New York: International Universities Press, 1962, 363-417.

Oring, Elliott, Ph.D. The Jokes of Sigmund Freud. Philadelphia: The University of Pennsylvania Press, 1984.

Rothman, Stanley, Ph.D. "Group Fantasies and Jewish Radicalism: A Psychodynamic Interpretation", Journal of Psychohistory, 6.2 (Fall, 1978)

Sheldon, William, M.D.,Ph.D. The Varieties of Temperament, A Psychology of Constitutional Differences. New York & London: Harper & Brothers, 1944.

Stein, Howard F., Ph.D. "Judaism and the Group-Fantasy of Martyrdom: The Psychodynamic Paradox of Survival Through Persecution", The Journal of Psychohistory, 6.2 (Fall, 1978).

Weidhorn, Manfred. "An Essay by Manfred Weidhorn." National Review, V XLIV, No. 5, March 16, 1992, S24-S28.

Wellhausen, Julius. Prolegomena to the History of Ancient Israel, Cleveland and New York: Meridian Books, 1957.

Whitman, Roy M., and Kaplan, Stanley M. "Clinical, Cultural and Literary Elaborations of the Negative Ego-Ideal." Comprehensive Psychiatry, V 9, No. 4, 1968, 358-371.

Williams, Daniel. "A Kinder, Gentler Zionism for Israel?", The Los Angeles Times, World Report Section, August 4, 1992

JEWS IV

William S. Horowitz, M.D. 2009

Common experiences with analysands and events on the current world scene, such as the money-changers' (bankers') ongoing crimes and the exposure of Madoff's Ponzi scheme, have led me to explore an area first touched on in several of my former essays: whether the *aggressive* Jew is not just an exception in that population but perhaps a regular feature of his society.

The Jew's persona as portrayed in popular literature and religious liturgy is too often proclaimed to be a victim, a passive, misunderstood, mistakenly prejudiced-against, poor, well-intentioned *schnook,* who only wants to get along with the rest of society if they will let him (as caricatured by Woody Allen). The description of him as a sharp untrustworthy manipulator is dismissed as envious or hateful slanderous prejudice by the *Goyim*. And the explanation of society's lack of acceptance of him as a product of his own diffidence, holding himself as *different* in so manifold ways, is accepted now by the Jew himself. And his role as a successful contemporary warrior is even lauded!

This formulation is salve to his conscience and a block to his self-understanding, a convenient rationalization to explain his difficult life vicissitudes in an ego-soothing way. And thus he goes about confident in his righteous victimhood and the world's evil, or at least unfairness, all the while supported by his religious mentors (thus insuring *their* usefulness).

A frequent feature of prolonged psychoanalysis of Jewish patients is the recovery of early memories and reactions to initial exposure to Jewish food, habits, and rituals as being *repellent,* only to be forgotten with the advent of the childhood amnesia to follow. This original impression of *ugliness* is perhaps later echoed in the adult publics perception of the behavior of the atavistic sect called Hassidim...but not regularly ascribed to socialized Jews, except by *committed anti-Semites*.

What have we here? Why should Jews be discriminated against, down through the ages yet, even after being re-admitted into societies which had previously banned them only to be re-expelled? Is this merely because they are different, because they are smart, because they claim to be morally superior, because they claim to sit at the grand leader's right hand, because of the Judas tale? Well, these may be true enough, and plausible enough to serve as psychic balms...but, are they really *sufficient* explanations?

Are you able to escape your inbred identification for a moment and look at yourself from the outside? If you were to undo all these reasons and to consider the proposition that the gentiles, the ones existing down through all ages and various societies, *consistently* had picked up something correctly about the Jews and were *rationally* reacting to it; what then? What are the odds they *all* were wrong? Is there something there for us to learn?

Professor Schlomo Sands of Tel-Aviv University has written about the pre-history of the Jews in the Holy Land, advancing the proposition that, contrary to popular myth that the tribes were flaccid victims of expulsion to wander in the desert, they were fierce warriors who drove *everyone else* out of the area before they were eventually subdued (perhaps reminiscent of today's Sabras conquering *five* attacking armies simultaneously). A visit to a Jewish Center gym will find no shortage of highly competitive athletes exercising their physical prowess, ... but their presence on professional athletic teams is striking by its paucity. Are star performers not wanted? Or are Jews simply not team players?

There are many examples of group aggressiveness which could be cited in contemporary and earlier history, but the classic one comes to mind in nineteenth century Germany. Then the Jews were historically perhaps the most successfully integrated into the larger society *ever* (perhaps by assimilation into the Christian milieu forming the Reform Temple); only in time to be perceived as being "too successful" and threatening to "take over", leading to the recrudescence of anti-Semitism and culminating eventually in the Mother of all programs.

Needless to post-script, perhaps the greatest historic *and on-going* example of the predatory Jew is Meyer (self-named) Rothschild and his genetic and ideological family of international bankers who, *to this day,* threaten the viability of our very own society! This is no hyperbole, Jewish reader: he is yours, and it behooves you to awaken to your heritage!

If this results in your becoming simultaneously angry and ashamed, less special and more humble, perhaps a bit more rational and a bit less chauvinistic, well, maybe that would be an acceptable outcome for a 21st century matured citizen of the world. That cultural *myths* may have survival value, there is no doubt; that they can outlive their usefulness may occur to some as well. Dispelling what may be the ancient romance about the Jewish tribe possibly could give more cogent effect to the cry, "Never Again!" *That* would seem to justify such an effort.

LETTER TO DR. BREINER

July 27th, 1991

Dear Dr. Breiner,

Thank you for your letter of July 8th, and for the time and effort you took to read and respond to my paper on Judaism. Since I solicited your opinion, I suppose the matter should rest there. Somehow, I am not content to leave your remarks unanswered.

I am aware and anticipated that those with strong religious convictions would have difficulty with the ideas I present, and I have no interest in engaging in a religious debate with you or anyone else. You are certainly entitled to your religious views, as am I. Furthermore, I am no religious scholar and am the first to admit it; therefore I have no problem with your criticism of my misunderstandings of Judaism or Christianity: there may well be doctrinal issues among others which I do not fully understand.

However, it was not my intention to explicate Jewish ritual or doctrine, but rather its psychology, and particularly its unconscious psychology. On this I feel on VERY firm ground after a long psychoanalytic experience with Jews and Christians alike, an experience I will gladly stack up against yours or anyone else's. In case you mistook me for a youngster, I am a semi-retired training and supervising analyst.

As for the criticism I propose unsubstantiated ideas, that is precisely the function of the paper, as a proposed hypothesis to be tested by other scholars and clinicians in the field. There is no need to prove an hypothesis, at least by the author proposing it, although I believe I present some compelling argument, judging by the reactions I have received from others.

Letter To Dr. Breiner

Your remark that the Seder is about freedom, not bondage, eludes me. How do you celebrate freedom from bondage without acknowledging the prior state? I could go on and on, but enough of this.

Your remark that I need further analysis is one which would have thrown me as a younger man, but now receive it with only mild irritation. I could equally claim that your apparent religious convictions could use more analytic investigation, too, but I wouldn't, for that would be an arrogant ad hominem argument. Let me only say, I have always found it curious that Jewish analysts I have known always attack analytically their Christian patients' religious identifications with a zeal matched only by their ignoring of their Jewish patients' identifications, with the curious resulting paradox of witnessing unabashed Orthodox observances amongst "well-analyzed" Jews. I see this as an example of a parochialism and chauvanism which only casts discredit on psychoanalysis.

As it so happens, my last analyst is still alive, and these are his comments about the paper (he is world famous as a clinician, writer, teacher, editor, and scientist): "It was an impressive work, thoughtful, scholarly, and closely reasoned. It is compact and compressed. I am sure that better authorities on this general subject than I will find much between these packed sentences to confirm, question, amplify and discuss."

I will be happy and satisfied if the real issues in the paper are thought about and discussed, let alone confirmed or refuted in times to come. All I ask is that you doff your rabbinical glasses long enough to consider the thesis. A Conservative cantor found the paper "compelling" after reconsidering it. A colleague of yours found it "persuasive". Yes, indeed, I am anti-Semitic, anti the bearded ones who think they are God and entitled to talk down to their subjects.

Sincerely,

William S. Horowitz, M.D.

LETTER TO DR. STEIN

August 4, 1991

Howard F. Stein, Ph.D.
Professor, Department of Family Medicine
The University of Oklahoma

Dear Howard,

I wanted to answer your letter of 24 July immediately, but I have been preoccupied since the day after I got it with my computer which got delayed in the shop for a whole week and then wouldn't work when it came home; just have it up and running tonight.

Your letter was exactly on target, and I am indebted to you for your unerring aim. Within 24 hours I had worked through whatever it was and realized the truth of your remark about fragmenting the work and myself. I understood that I have been writing on aspects of only one issue for all these years, narcissism, which has also preoccupied me clinically, and that the pieces do all belong together. So I am going to proceed as methodically as I can to follow your experienced prescription and see what happens. Thank you, again. You are quite the mentor, indeed. As a fringe benefit, this realization was accompanied by a great relief of indecision, elation, and a sense of longitudinal purpose and wholeness to my work and me. (One of the pieces I have to decide about including is autobiographical, tracing the origins of this interest.) Only to have technology or perverse fate slow me down just when the iron was hot!

It is well for me to remember your other caution about the built-in resistance to this topic of Judaism, like its substrate, narcissism, which I tend to underestimate in professional audiences. In 1964 I gave a long paper before our Institute which was so well received that 50 colleagues asked for a series of evening seminars on it...we spent three evenings going over it in detail, during which, believe it or not, not a single question was asked!

More contemporaneously and of more direct interest to you, I answered DeMause's (and Breiner's) objections to the Judaism paper, and in the process made reference to you, (which correspondence I'd like to share with you but am afraid it would be too great an imposition on your time) only to hear by return mail he will reconsider it and send it out to other readers if American Imago rejects it. So...! The squeaking axle gets the grease?

I didn't mean to spend so much time on myself, but to convey how helpful you have been. Then I got your beautiful paper. It is a literary pearl. And a joy to share your intimate thoughts and feelings via this perspective on your life. And Chicago, Frederic Stock, Rumania, violin, and walking all resonate with personal experiences of my own, allowing me to feel a tiny bit akin to you and your father. I have not read all of your work, naturally...yet. But I do hope if you haven't already done so that you consider a longer autobiography, for it seems to me, indeed in your hands, a compelling vehicle for communicating insights the texture of which I can't imagine being conveyed in any other way.

I see also that besides a common (but different) heritage of Judaism that we share, that we both have a lot of father in us, a rare and precious commodity, don't you think, which makes for instant rapport between like kinds and instant repulsion between unlike ones...the unmagnetic effect. It is such a personal pleasure to me to assist young physicians (and homosexuals for that matter) in recovering their own closet masculinity, which is so beleaguered these days. I had the thought that maybe in researching some of the blue-collar groups you have worked with, this welcome quality is in greater supply and adds an interest to the research. Do you think so? Could we call this a 20th century father-hunger?

Howard, you have set me on the right track, offered me company, and now friendship. I don't know what I have done to deserve this, but I am appreciative and grateful, and still puzzled by its rarity amongst professionals like ourselves. Have you found in your work at the medical school that doctors make lousy friends? I continually get this impression and have some ideas about it. In fact, that would make a good paper, for I have worked chiefly with them these last 20 years. The previous twenty was spent in "Hollywood" with all the creative artists. Maybe one day we can visit over drinks and acquaint ourselves better.

Hope you have a cool and restful, relatively, summer.

THE SIGNIFICANCE OF THE PERIOD OF 4 YEARS IN THE EDUCATIONAL PROCESS

It is a remarkable fact that the figure of 4 years recurs with uncanny regularity in the area of education or influence-ability of one person by another.

All manner of curricula are organized on this basis: elementary and junior high (together make 8), high school, college, professional schools, gymnasium (8), psychoanalytic seminars, etc. I am informed that in Britain breaks in the educational continuum occur at ages 6, 10, 14, and 18. Most interesting is the data revealed by Lewin and Ross: that the period from matriculation to graduation of psychoanalytic candidates proves out to be 8 years, and that the average duration of training analysis of 773 hours at a frequency of 4.2 hours per week yields (assuming a working year of 46 weeks) 4 years. (Cf. Szasz' article on the significance of the period of 5 years in psychoanalytic training and immigration.)

We elect our president for a term of 4 years Other terms of office are variants of this module: 2 and 6. Likewise, the modal period of military enlistment is 4 years. It is claimed in pop psychology that the crucial year for a marriage is the 4th. Trade apprenticeships typically last 4 years. The average household mortgage is held 6 years before the average move takes place. It would be relevant to gather statistics in other "demographic" areas, for example, of prison sentences, junior executive job shifts, transfers of non-tenured university instructors, etc., to see if this same periodicity exists there, too.

Somewhere in his early writings Freud makes reference to the age of 8 as a crucial one; I cannot find the reference yet. But consider this passage in "Three Contributions...":

"There seems no doubt that germs of sexual impulses are already present in the new-born child and that these continue to develop for a time, but are then overtaken by a progressive process of suppression; this in turn is itself interrupted by periodical advance in sexual development or may be held up by individual peculiarities. Nothing is known for certain concerning the regularity and periodicity of this oscillating course of development. It seems, however, that the sexual life of children usually emerges in a form accessible to observation round about the third or fourth year of life."

"It is during this period of total or only partial latency that are built up the mental forces which are later to impede the course of the sexual instinct and, like dams, restrict its flow – disgust, feelings of shame and the claims of aesthetic and moral ideals. One gets an impression from civilized children that the construction of these dams is a product of education, and no doubt education has much to do with it. But in reality this development is organically determined and fixed by heredity, and it can occasionally occur without any help at all from education. Education will not be trespassing beyond its appropriate domain if it limits itself to following the lines which have already been laid down organically and to impressing them somewhat more clearly and deeply."

According to Jones, Freud's period of active collaboration with Breuer started in 1892; 1896 marked the switch from Breuer to Fliess, and 1900 the end with Fliess. More difficult to determine was the period of self-analysis, but on page 320 is a reference to 3 or 4 years, on page 327, 4 or 5 years.

Can it be that there is a fairly regular cycle in normals and neurotics approximating 4 years in duration, during which their influence-ability (and transference) progressively diminishes as their own sexuality emerges, at the end of which cycle new parental surrogates must be found with which to re-work the (Oedipal) problems at a higher level?

Is it possible to find and define such a cycle in the following sequence: primary Oedipal period with parents; early latency (to 4th grade) with teachers; late latency (to 8th grade) with a shift to other parental figures, perhaps parents of contemporaries; adolescence (high school) in which an attempt is made to simultaneously come to grips with new parental surrogates and to do away altogether with authority figures in a peer society; then college; then post-graduate or professional school; (now to use an example) internship and residency; then training analysis (4) and seminars (4) in a matrix of 8 years?

All manner of questions arise, and the ramifications seem endless; a few follow. Is there a deeper factor at work in the coming to a close of an analysis (or for that matter, a phase of raising a child, or a relationship with an adult)? Is there validity to the subjective experience of losing one's power or influence over one's patient? Are our explanations of unresolved resistances, increasing success and gratification of the patient, loss of the analyst's interest, and so on, and our recommendations for more life experience, consolidation, and completing the work with another analyst...are these mere rationalizations in the face of some unmitigating instinctual flux?

Does the course of an object relationship follow a natural evolution, the absence of which marks disturbance? Is this the hallmark of fixation? One can maintain an object relationship without fixation by entering a new phase (normal evolution), but can this be done without the addition of new objects? Does the psychotic suffer from a "complete fixation" in which the time element is lost, past and present merging, with infantile objects perceived ubiquitously? What bearing does the object relationship have on suppression of instinctual flux... and vice versa? Is acting-out a half-way station to this phenomenon? Is normal transference a quarter-way station?

What about our old friend, repetition compulsion? Is it there, and can it really be modified by analysis? Do we invoke the rule of abstinence for rational reasons...and then proceed to progressively permit its transgression for rational reasons, or are we repeating a pattern from our ontogenetic and phylogenetic past?

What about interpretations? Or is it a question of our not interfering with, and correctly keeping pace with a naturally evolving object-relationship? Do we lead a patient, or follow him? Are our interventions really communications that we understand what he is expressing and can go on? Are the insights his or ours?

What of the role of the ego in all of this? If we truly reclaim areas of the id for the ego, perhaps we must recognize that in spite of this reclamation, the instincts retain their supremacy. How else explain this surprising and prosaic skeleton in the closet of psychoanalytic treatment and training? (The cultural pattern argument does not go deep enough, and begs the question.)

SPECULATIONS
DRAFT OF A WORK IN PROGRESS

William S. Horowitz, M.D.

This will be an attempt to describe and define the characteristics and differences between the holders of liberal and conservative political positions. Since the subject matter is so invested with emotion, itself an interesting phenomenon, an attempt will be made to use value-neutral terms and concepts.

Perhaps the starting point ought to be the aims of the two groups. In a general way and according to common understanding, the liberal wants to liberate, free, move on, evolve, or revolt against the felt limitations and constraints of a political system in order to improve what is felt to be malfunctioning in that system; the conservative, on the other hand, wants to save and return to previously held values which he feels have been abandoned in an ill-advised move toward "improvement".

In this common view, the liberal is forward-looking, the conservative backward-looking (both terms easily capable of being loaded with pejorative value). This brings us to its corollary: that the liberal outlook is typical of youth, conservative of age. When described in this way, one can entertain the relative symmetry of the positions around a neutral centerpoint, and the absence of any intrinsic relative superiority or inferiority of either.

There are a whole host of elaborations that can be made about each of these political attitudes, but they will be foregone for the moment in the interests of further speculation at this level. If each of these positions can be naturally fitted into a time-of-life axis, can there ever be any absolute or heuristic value placed upon them, any more than saying it is better/worse to be younger/older? The issue might then be to consider their relative value, their appropriateness, at certain points on this axis and under certain (political) conditions. This might imply, additionally, a natural progression from one position to the other over time, and the possibility of interference in that progression, introducing the concepts of regression, fixation, and pre-maturity in an otherwise natural progression.

Now comes the first value judgment: we could say the first position is immature but normal (modal) at a youthful stage of life, residual or fixated at a mature age; just as the second position is abnormal (pre-mature) at an early age but modal at a mature one. Here we come up against an assumption that common sense and usage compels: that these political attitudes are indeed age-related, in the broad, which I will not further argue at this point. Indeed, does it not seem unusual, un-modish, or abnormal for the younger to be backward looking, the older forward? The younger conservative seems progeric, the older liberal fixated, nicht wahr?

Now that we have become somewhat comfortable with placing the political philosophies on an age continuum, let us further elaborate on the contextual details of each.

The liberal or youth, interested as he is in resisting the status quo or even regressive pull of his society, yearns to be free of all constraint, regulation, direction, assumptions, or external forces in general. He is therefore anti-what is, pro-what ought to be, rebellious, idealistic, attacking and destroying for the good cause. He is by nature aggressive, by feeling entitled, by conscience justified: ergo, there are few restraints on his attacks on the social structure, which aim to re-make it into idealized images. He identifies with all of mankind, particularly the oppressed like himself, and fancies his complaints and solutions to be novel and unique (experiencing himself and therefore his feelings as brand new, not testing them against history which would be backward-looking).

Without the defeats of experience, he is optimistic, indeed omnipotently so, that any goal can be reached if only steadfastly held. Therefore he is loyal to his calling and confreres, and persistent even, perhaps, in the face of contrary evidence. Also without the benefit of experience and with his associated tendency to think globally in idealized images, he does not discriminate between the good which works and the bad that needs elimination, tending toward global replacement of total societal institutions instead of modifications of existing ones. He thinks in absolute terms of good and bad, allies himself with the good and attacks the bad with unmitigated, righteous zeal. He also brooks no interference or advice from the more experienced, who are viewed as personal adversaries to be vanquished.

The quality of his aggression, like its targets, tends to be global and therefore indiscriminate, impulsive and uncontrolled, explosive and "hot": he prefers the blunderbuss, the broadside, the weapon of mass destruction, the un-aimable weapon. The expression could be thought of as pre-genital and mother-identified, the vehicle often the arts, the liberal arts, particularly the performing arts, tolerant of deviation with the objective often of bringing about massive change in the status of conditions in the society. Authority is equated with "bad", rebellion with "good" by these (women and children) unempowered members of society.

We have then the picture of the liberal as younger, energetic, aggressive, forward-looking, rebellious (against authority), without assets, socialistic, inclusive, power-seeking, entitled, idealistic, destroying (killing) and re-constructive, justified, optimistic, omnipotent, polarized, persistent, unlearning, enemy-making, loyal, zealous, and perhaps female-identified.

The mature conservative, having the benefits of time and experience and hind-sight, likely is enjoying the fruits of his labors, relishing the enjoyable social institutions and his place in them, satisfied and perhaps contented, and is power-retaining, reminiscing about the "good old days" and wanting to return to or save them, passive, realistic, ambivalent, pessimistic, adapting and modifying rather than replacing but altogether resistant to change, conserving, discriminating, excluding, learning, sifting of values, friend-making, conciliatory, not righteous but accepting, nondestructive, perhaps fatigued, and possibly male-identified.

His aggression is likely to be controlled and "cool", carefully and discriminately aimed, "phallic" in nature, preferring as a vehicle the gun, the rifle, the barbed mot. He tends to be father-identified and is comfortable with the arts of the martial variety. He would tend to be the defender rather than the initiator of aggression, intolerant of change, protecting and preserving of developed arrangements, values, and authority, being the empowered one in the society.

The older conservative, in political terms, is thus the "have" and only has everything to lose; the younger liberal is the "have not" and has nothing to lose and only something to gain. Ergo, by nature, the liberal is the aggressive attacker, the conservative the passive defender. When, in the course of time, the younger liberal acquires that which the older conservative has already accomplished, he in turn becomes the (envied) older conservative. Pictured or defined in this way, these political positions are transformed into psychological stages in life, and, as such, perhaps subject to more rational discourse.

Conservatives, being older, look to themselves; liberals, being younger, look to their idealized parents for satisfaction of their needs, representing a child/parent relationship. Therefore, socialism is the arrangement of youth, individualism (capitalism) the arrangement of maturity.[1] The conservative feels degraded by socialistic arrangements, the liberal cheated by individualistic ones (of his just due, perhaps, in a deprived and therefore fixated childhood). The young capitalist/individualist perhaps was sufficiently parented and modeled to immediately have conservatism as his aim. Contrast with the incomplete self-object separation (differentiation) of the liberal, which results in group-think, the suppression of individualism, and the undue prolongation of dependence. Perhaps the struggle between political classes is ultimately over the necessity of growing up.

Related to the above considerations are the use of particular defense mechanisms. The incomplete self-object separation in the liberal tends to the use of projective mechanisms, (mis-)identifying his own aggressive characteristics in his opponent which serves as a provocation, tending to induce the unwanted aggression in his object. In addition, this inherent aggression is usually accompanied by an idealistic denial of its existence, constituting an egregious transparent hypocrisy that additionally introduces provocation into the attempted dialogue[2]. The liberal, by nature, is the agent provocateur, the conservative (parent) the flummoxed victim, left sputtering in impotent rebuttal. A true dialogue is therefore difficult to engineer between these polarities. Not a true observation, but the liberal is prone to see the conservatives as in conspiracy against him. The usual truth in the accusation lies in the consensus that undoubtedly exists among the audience watching his machinations (which is not to deny the historical existence of political and business combinations in the forms of dictatorships and cartels). It is as in the young delinquent who complains that the whole society is against him.

There is a suggestion here of a natural antagonism between the young and the old, and by extension, between the liberal and the conservative. This antagonism or rivalry can assume the proportions of an armed camp, with the implicit threat of annihilation if one's position is not successfully defended. Here perhaps lies the explanation for the heavy investment of emotion in these philosophical political positions: they represent narcissistic positions, or self-defending ones (which also necessitate the erection of opposites or enemies).

How to account for the exceptions, the younger conservative and the older liberal? We have used the terms pre-maturity and fixation to describe them, but what does that say except that they are occurring at an age-inappropriate or age-unusual stage? If we consider the time-of-life axis as connoting a gradual accumulation of experience (?and wisdom) plus a gradual diminishment of energy, then these terms are judged to have value, or more properly, counter-balancing values. The younger liberal is energetic, the older conservative wiser; the younger conservative is then energetic and wise, the older liberal is experienced but still hopeful. I submit that many of our most creative writers and artists were at the extremes of the age axis (the tails of the bell-shaped curve) when they produced their most significant contributions, either unusually young or old for that activity. Perhaps these are the exceptions which "prove the rule".

Does this mean we should look to our exceptions for guidance? Perhaps, but the general implication here is that these two positions are not likely to mesh or merge, but remain polarized and alternating in their perpetual struggle for dominance in the society. And perhaps in the larger picture, these counter-balancing forces constitute a natural dynamic equilibrium in the society that provides both stability and the possibility of buffered movement in the social body. Political systems or their agents which seek to exploit the tensions in a society for the purposes of destabilizing that society and revolutionizing it find ready if unwitting accomplices in the liberal/radical group, the "useful fools" of Marx and Lenin.

This time axis by no means exhausts the sources of an individual's political affiliations. There are at least two more obvious ones: his individual history, and his individual psychology. As for the former, families, socio-economic classes, geographic areas, religious affiliations, professions, and other specific factors are sources of identifications that go into an individual's composite identity and thus his political temperament. In similar fashion, his unique personality characteristics may match singular or combinations of attributes in a political position that may attract or make it congenial to him. We have thus named at least three major sources of an individual's politics: his age, his history, and his personality. This reminds us that we should include a fourth, a temporal or circumstantial factor, which may dictate a political philosophy over-riding his natural bent and cause him to side with those with whom he is not entirely identified. (As we have it, "Politics makes strange bed-fellows".) Needless to add, one individual's political philosophy may be a mixture of the two polar positions regarding different departments of the society, but the "well-tempered" eclectic is a rare bird, indeed.

In this view, the argument of natural superiority by adherents of either position with its attendant contempt for the other is an egregious conceit, more characteristic of children with their team loyalties than thoughtful adults pondering the problems of their troubled society. And doubly unseemly when proffered by presumptuous pundits politicizing their professional pronouncements with personal proclivities. But, as discussed elsewhere (see my paper on Power), the choosing of an external government (written at the time of the 1992 national election) is indeed a regressive practice when contrasted with the exercise of one's own internal governance, and so perhaps the regressive phenomena should not surprise us. The choosing of our national president, then, is not so very distant in our psychological lives from the choosing of our high school class president.

And here in this American institution of erecting a youthful leader to challenge the established monarchy we revisit the old Revolutionary Oedipal struggle and its centennial re-edition in the Union North / Rebel South battle, that finds its continuing echo in the liberal / conservative one of today. ["Plus ca change, plus c'est la meme chose."]

In America, the liberal position has most often found its home in the Democratic party [3](although in earlier times the Republicans called themselves the liberals), the conservative position in the Republican; in Britain, the Labor party and the Tory party, respectively. Here can be seen the social class distinction between the workers and the landed gentry or Royalists, reflected in the House of Commons and the House of Lords, the predecessor to our classes of demos and Publicans and our institutions of House of Representatives and Senate.

The extremes of these positions are known as the radical liberals and the reactionary conservatives. These terms, of course, carry a certain emotional loading of opprobrium inferring excess, and are subject to even further manipulation, distortion, and outright falsification for political and propaganda purposes, as in the identification of radical Communism recently in the Soviet and China as reactionary. But, in part this "mis"-naming reflects our earlier thesis, that of the normal aging of the population and the shift from what was originally radically liberal (heterodoxy) to what is reactionary conservative (orthodoxy or establishment).

Since the seating in the French assembly, it is said, the practice has spread of identifying the liberal with the "left", the conservative with the "right", which has fascinating etymological and preconscious inferences.

Speculations Draft Of A Work In Progress

The implications of left = left out and sinister (L., sinistra), right = might, correct, establishment cannot have escaped your attention [4]. Usually these adjectives are used with the noun "wing" to denote the extensions on the body of the polity, with the further unspoken implication that the central mass is neither.

As one example of a professional "bias" toward a particular political philosophy, medicine has always been identified with conservatism, with the outstanding exception of one specialty, psychiatry and psychoanalysis, which is the sanctuary of liberalism, often activist liberalism [5]. Is this the product of a humanist philosophy? Probably not, for there is no reason to believe psychiatrists are any more humanistic than other physicians. Is this a product of the historical European source of the field? Perhaps. Or is this a reflection of the fact that the specialty is heavily Jewish (and has been called the "Jewish Science" by its detractors), and that Jews as a political group are well-known to be radical liberal [6]. I think here lies the most compelling explanation, and with it, the illustration of an ethnic political philosophy.

The age progression earlier described for individuals can also be applied to larger social institutions, such as religions, for instance. The Jewish religion could be thought of as radical liberal as it broke with earlier pantheistic beliefs to proclaim its tenet of monotheism. In time it became the conservator of this and other beliefs, the protector of orthodoxy, as the Christian religion broke away in liberating revolt.

This was followed in time by Catholicism becoming the establishment or conservator, particularly in central and southern Europe, where eventually its political power led the way to corrupt, loosened, or liberalized practices, enabling the Eastern Orthodox Church to separate itself to the right to challenge the hegemony of the establishment. Likewise Protestantism in its turn several centuries later broke away to the right in its rebellious heterodoxy, only in turn to become the establishment, particularly in America.

The latter two movements, like what is happening in contemporary Iran and other Islamic societies, including also segments of our own

Christian American one, were and are returns to religious fundamentalism, or reactionary to perceived excesses in the other direction. The analogous development within the Jewish religion is the rise of a particular form of Orthodoxy (Hasidic) in the face of what it perceives to be excessive dilution in westernized Reform Judaism. This illustrates that both right and left can revolt against each other, or, better, that excesses in either direction are reacted to by the rise of opposing forces, rendering in sum a dynamic stabilizing. The term reactionary is thus not limited to conservative positions but equally well applies to liberal ones.

The "gridlock" in American government recently popularized, by inference a failure in the democratic process, could be thought of quite oppositely as the successful buffering of the body politic through the extension and empowerment of the voting public preventing the retention of power by any one faction. But, it equally well could be conceptualized as the grabbing of power away from the electorate by the career politicians and entrenched interests, thus introducing a dis-equilibrium between the power-givers and the power-seekers. We could say that what is gridlocked is the power or effectiveness of government, what may be dis-enfranchised is the electorate.

However, even within the power-seekers a dynamic shift has occurred, as the recent election has seen a 70 year-old president be replaced by a 40 year-old one. This would argue for a continuing metamorphosis within a dynamic equilibrium, something the founding fathers unarguably would smile in satisfaction about. So, while as politically sentient individuals we cheer the popular success of our own point of view and similarly feel disappointment about its refutation, as members of a society of others we may find consolation in the continuing vital maintenance and evolution of the polity, contrasted against the dire predictions of "the end" voiced by the extremists.

The extremists thus by definition are of one mind only and see their extinction in the refutation of their policies: they are thus narcissistic. By contrast, the absolute centrist without any individual identification, the body between the wings who is known as the "chicken", would be as pathological as the extremist in his identity-less-ness.

The adherents of the right and left, the "centrists" of either party, are more balanced and can admit the existence of others with countervailing points of view (requiring separate object cathexis and the toleration of ambivalence) and are thus both more mature. Having their own point of view but respectful of the existence of others' perhaps is the mark of political as well as emotional adulthood. This tolerance, this American political virtue, this capacity to include many which enables our unique and distinguishing society, cannot help but be linked to the Christian charity and tolerance practiced by the Protestant majority, and stands in sharp contrast to all the other more-or-less homogeneous and exclusionary societies on earth.

The mature member of the polity is thus neither liberal nor conservative to the exclusion of the other, but is identified with his position while fully aware of and respectful of others. Because of the significance of aging in the process of emotional maturation, probably the conservative is statistically usually more mature than the liberal...but likewise, the liberal statistically usually more energetic, hopeful, visionary, and an agent for change. The political process needs both, of course, as does the society need young and old. There is no place for smugness in this formulation.

We referred earlier to the omnipotence of the young liberal, and the acceptance of constituted authority (or "reality") in the older conservative. This is one reflection of the psychological maturation that has gone on in the course of time: the relinquishment of one's personal sense of power and self-absorption in the gradual acknowledgement of outside beings and forces of greater magnitude. This shift and recognition can refer to human authority, the irresistibility of impersonal forces of nature, and/or the superimposition of these two ideas into the conception of a deity. In this perspective, the child is the god, the adult acknowledges the father and respects/worships the god.

Here we come upon the explanation of the Jew's political liberalism, for he is well known to be atheistic, in contrast to almost all other known religions. (How the Jew nominally worships "the God of the Jews" when he is religious, which in increasing numbers he is not, and at the same time harbors within himself the deepest doubt of the existence of any deity, is a separate fascinating subject.) By extension and analogy, does not the young political liberal also feel he has the knowledge, the power, and the mandate to punish all evil, destroy his enemies, and remake society in his own vision if not image? This is the sine qua non of the liberal's omnipotent political outlook, betraying his identification with the god himself. The conservative is thus viewed as thwarting this objective, a sworn enemy of his powers, and in need of destruction.

Here we have but one aspect of the struggle between the psychological forces of progression and regression, the struggle over growing up, to which all the human race is heir by virtue of its prolonged dependence, which is enabled by the social non-necessity of autonomous functioning. In no other species, probably, is there such a struggle over the issue of maturation, either internally or between the members of that society. Can we speculate whether that is why there are no politics in other species, no struggle of one group to have power over another? Elm trees and fruit flies merely maturate, insensibly following the inborn dictates of their nature in a totally "natural" and unimpeded progression. Human beings fight it all the way, fighting the internal and external forces that impel that movement. Chief among the latter are the figure of the father, that representative of the "reality" of the outside world. The acknowledgement of the father, religious or secular as the case may be, the acceptance of the limits to the exercise of one's own power over things and people, is thus the hallmark of maturation from youth to manhood, and from liberal to conservative in the political sphere.

Yes, here is a value introduced into the argument, and an important one, for it corresponds to the state of the public body which is overwhelmingly conservative in its outlook and presumably experienced and mature. There is no equivalence of value in these two sides of the debate when viewed from the psychological angle, only when considered in detached abstraction. So, in spite of attempting a value-neutral examination of the political polarities, I am forced to conclude that politics does indeed center on the urge to exert power over fellow beings, and that it reflects the ongoing intrapsychic and interpsychic struggle over maturation.

That this struggle is distinctively human, that it will be ultimately lost, that we as a society indulge this destructive struggle far beyond its experimental (playful) reach, all these seem commonplace; yet if we contemplate the opposite, the early compelling of reconciliation with reality, we know we can produce a non-human apolitical robotic society which is equally undesirable. The exercise of politics can then be said to "humanize" society, an observation that you will recognize has rarely been voiced. In this view liberals should be tolerated and their suggestions appreciated, but they must never, ever be allowed to take control of the polity, or the family. But they will no doubt remind us that the conservatives should not be allowed it, either.

In a feature article in the Chicago Tribune Magazine of January 16th, 1994 entitled "What Price Correctness; Dumbocracy in America", Harvard English professor and artistic director of the American Repertory Theatre Robert Brustein observes, "In his preface to 'The Liberal Imagination', Lionel Trilling quoted Goethe's remark that liberals have no ideas, they have only sentiments. Obviously, little has changed in the intervening years. What has changed is the virtual monopoly on ideas by the conservative camp (and this from a liberal author!). Trilling had cautioned liberals to take as their motto, 'Lord, enlighten thou my enemies', because intelligent opposition was the only way he saw to develop a sensible body of liberal thought. He did not foresee a time when the opposition would dominate thinking, while liberals sat impotent, mired in sentiment or paralyzed with guilt."

---

1   Thus also the liberals tend to band together in groups, famously found in large population centers in political action organizations called "machines" which for all of history have dominated American metropolitan politics, a phenomenon totally foreign

to conservatives. Liberal constituencies are found then in the large cities of this country, as well as in the immigrant, minority, organized labor, civil servant, some professional (legal), and impoverished clusters wherever they appear.

2	See my paper "Toward a Unifying Conception of Narcissism" in which the primary process discharge speech of youth contrasted with the secondary process communication of maturity is described.

3	The Democratic party has practiced "machine politics" in its history in all the metropoli, run by a "boss" and ward leaders, who support their constituency with money and expect votes in return, a powerful source of generational loyalty to the party and accounting for the prevalence of liberal philosophies in the big cities, minorities, and the poor. It is a reproduction of the parent/child relationship and generates an understandable enduring faithfulness through the generations and centuries. The Republicans have no such organizations nor do they perceive the need for them. The blind loyalty to the "party" by Negroes, to Roosevelt by Jews, the resistance to modifying his legacy of Social Security, all can be seen as products of this unthinking faith.

4	cf. Patrick Buchanan's book title, "Right From the Start".

5	Hence the authors cited earlier.

6	cf. my paper, "Let My People Go!"

WASP-A PROTESTANT DISEASE, AMERICAN GOTHIC, OR THE STATE OF WASPISHNESS.

William S. Horowitz, M.D.

The idea for this paper arose during the long course of attempted therapy and analysis with a series of patients having certain character traits in common, and was crystallized during an informal discussion with a respected Gentile colleague, who responded to my complaints of frustration in trying to understand a particularly difficult clinical case with (words to the effect) "Why, she's just your average "WASP". The title "Protestant Disease" is meant in both senses, both as a psychological illness Protestants seem susceptible to, and the consequent notion of the religious culture as an historical institutionalization of a founding individual's characterological pathology.

Knowing full well the difficulties and dangers of attempting a religious and ethnic character typology, I am impelled to proceed never-the-less by the continuing influx of similar data and the clinical challenge of understanding them. The focus in this paper will not be on tracing fascinating historical, cross-religious, sociological, and contemporary American political issues, though interesting points of departure will be indicated, but rather on an attempted descriptive delineation and discussion of prominent dynamic and structural features of my prototypical Protestant patient's character and functioning.

The ideas presented here have been gathered over a period of some thirty-five years of psychoanalytic practice and over sixty-five years of living and working with a predominantly Christian clientele and culture (to be sure, through the eyes of a non-Protestant observer). They have been gathered against considerable personal resistance and are presented in a spirit of scientific inquiry as an outgrowth of the author's continuing interest in the problem of narcissism and its derivative, character. The ideas are offered with considerable trepidation, for they could provide ammunition for unscientific abuse as well as material for psychic defense, and with the expectation that like portraits can and will be developed for the prototypical white Catholic, Jew (now completed), and Negro in turn, the other significant religious-ethnic groups in our American culture (as of the '70's).

Needless to say, the author is no theological scholar, but would welcome information from such sources which might confirm or contradict his observations and fill in his psychoanalytic premises.

It should be needless to disclaim but unfortunately necessary that this is a composite character study which reflects no individual real person, but as a generalization and mosaic attempts to include data gathered from many. By the same token, there are obviously many exceptions to this picture among Protestant patients, possibly even the majority, the study of whom should prove especially valuable at pin-pointing the etiological factors which may account for the difference. I have seen the identical picture of intimacy-lessness in both Jews and Catholics in instances where they shared in common mothers who had been raised in an orphanage.

Especially fascinating to me has been to trace the patient's struggle as a child of mixed parentage; mothers, when Protestant, seem to be the key force influencing the child. I believe my clinical experience has sampled a broad range of denominations, but the most over-represented of all the sects has been the patient raised by a Christian Scientist mother. These patients seem to reflect the broad range of character configurations found amongst many of the denominations.

To repeat, this is a study of a composite group of Protestant patients I have worked with clinically, the purpose of which is to try to understand what contribution the WASP culture made to their individual pathologies, and pari-passu, what illumination the individuals throw on the nature of the culture.

I

The patients who are the focus of this investigation all have to varying degrees similar problems in the areas of talking, eating, eliminating, touching, affectivity, empathy, human relations, socializing, pleasure and satisfaction. The therapeutic situation seems to present a unique and painful challenge to them. They present themselves at interview in a stiff and formal manner, often strikingly over-dressed for the occasion long after others would have relaxed into informality. Talking seems always to be difficult and silence easier (taciturn, like Coolidge). Speech is halting, spare, flat, ungenerous, often loud (reflecting subjective interpersonal long-distance), sometimes hostile, and the content and scope of the ideation superficial, reflecting an active intellectual inhibition. Conveying little or no emotion, it is unmoving and boring and difficult to empathize with. Ideas are glib, prosaic, and at the level of "newspaper mentality". Cliches replace original or deep concepts.

Superficially, the patient seems empty of inner life or rigorously defended against it. Instinctual discharge is usually directed somatically, in action, or into isolated intellectualized thinking. Loving and giving impulses are rigidly controlled, unspontaneous, and only ritually released on ceremonial occasions such as Christmas, along with otherwise strongly-tabooed expressions of need and want. Elimination and impulse regulation is also marked by over-control which seems to sustain a tenuous self-esteem. "Giving in" to feelings, urges, or another's expectations is accompanied by exquisite humiliation (the shame of incontinence).

Eating is performed with a similar lack of enthusiasm (as is the taking in of the analyst's interventions), almost as a grudging obligation to sustain life but with no obvious pleasure or satisfaction. They often have a childhood and continuing history of being picky eaters and tend toward reactions of mistrust to new offerings and experiences, particularly if generous and warm. Family mealtimes are generally a disaster; they can be almost totally decathected, ritualized or fragmented, mirroring the early mother-infant feeding disturbance which sooner or later is given up as a failure. There is an association built between feeding and discomfort (the bristly-nipple phenomenon).

These patients often give the history of no conscious recollection of having been embraced by either parent, who are excused as being "undemonstrative", and many manifest a touching phobia on multiple inner and outer

Wasp-a Protestant Disease, American Gothic, Or The State Of Waspishness.

levels (or an episodically-driven type of "stimulus hunger" which looks like sexual impulsivity). In addition to the usual physical touching phobias, there may be a functionally selective deafness, eye-aversion, affective distancing (lack of empathy), and intellectual sequestering (provincialism). The intrapsychic distancing between parts yields a dynamic dis-integration or insulation or isolation or splitting. All of these phenomena directly reflect and repeat the deliberate (though) unconscious actual interruptions in earliest mother-infant contacts, the deprivation in the primary symbiotic fusion experiences. Eye contact is particularly phobically avoided in some, several turning their faces 180o away in conversation!

Conscious memories of masturbation may also be lacking, and the being out of touch with how they themselves and others "feel" is striking. Thus their own affectivity and empathy is grossly defective, which, combined with their intellectual inhibition, gives rise to a pseudo-stupidity, derisively labeled in Yiddish "Goische Kopf". Their disturbed and unintegrated primary process functioning and resistance to creativity is also often reflected in a lack of a sense of esthetics: being tone and rhythm deaf, color and design blind, with a preference for colorless gray, non-ambiguous hard-edge design.

In a larger sense, they are "artless" and unintellectual, lacking the sublimatory capacities consequent to their defective primary symbiotic experience, though they share vicariously the cultural sublimations of their religion. Thus, Bible reading, church attendance, and practicing religious rituals as well as appreciating religious art, philosophy and music can constitute, for some, the whole of their cultural existence. In the extreme, a regressive relationship with the mothering church becomes the all-encompassing experience, to the exclusion of interpersonal relationships and an individual psychology, thereby replicating the missed and wished for fusion experience with mother. In non-religious, present-generation people, this same relationship can take place with any group, institution, activity, or topical philosophy (cult), and is readily replaceable by any other (identity by membership and belief). Even the devout are able to switch their ministers and houses of worship like a new hat, to be "in style".

Affects typically are somatized; emerge incontinently to be experienced briefly and shamefully and then impulsively acted upon or re-suppressed; or denied which gives rise to an hysteric-appearing indifference. Pain, especially psychic pain, is stoically endured and needs are spartanly suppressed: "Stiff upper-lip, ya' know". Pleasure arouses anxiety and feelings of badness and must be carefully rationed and paid for. Satisfaction, of one's own needs by another, is rigorously avoided and unacknowledged.

Almost none of the patients in my series was overtly religious and practicing their faith, and generally minimized the importance of their childhood training or belief which typically did not endure into adulthood. Almost all gave a history of a parent actively practicing a religion, usually the mother. Where parents represented an interfaith marriage or one religious and one not, the Protestant mother's influence seemed the stronger. All the patients came with the complaint of, or evidenced, serious problems in sustaining an intimate heterosexual relationship and gave the impression of general immaturity, sometimes downright childishness. Neither neurotic nor psychotic syndromes were in the foreground (i.e., they represented character disorders) but mechanisms of both, of course, were employed.

II

The primary fixation point appeared to have been oral, and the trauma to have been an abrupt and sustained weaning from oral gratification with a compensatory premature (and defective) self and ego development propelled into the anal phase, giving rise to a predominately reactive, denying, and synthetic character structure. Because of its enforced premature separation from the mother, the child is left not having undergone the normal symbiotic phase and narcissistic resolution, evidencing many manifestations of arrested and incomplete individuation, narcissistic features (among which a quest for power and overvaluation of appearances, looking good and being good-looking, are prominent), and a false or pseudo-self.

The early trauma also predisposes to somatization reactions, addictions, and ego and character deformations, rather than psychoneurotic ones, hence the illness equals the character. The two most predominant symptoms are the incapacity for interpersonal intimacy and the abuse of alcohol, which serves multiple functions (vide infra).

As a group the patients in my series did not represent hopeful treatment prospects, at least with expressive talking psychotherapies, lacking both the psychic contents and expressive capacities, as well as empathy and psychological-mindedness and capacity for sustained object-relationships which analysis requires. In addition, the deprivation of the psychoanalytic situation too closely replicated the conditions at home and was intolerable. Supportive feeding therapies may offer possibilities of leading to more, however (of which Alcoholics Anonymous, representing a sustained and enforced family relationship may provide a helpful model). Their deep oral rage, destructive envy, and resistances to giving, receiving, closeness and contact, make them especially susceptible to negative therapeutic reactions, the most common acute form of which is the abrupt souring toward and leaving of treatment in the face of an apparent good working relationship and evidence of mounting positive transference, often with a verbalized stinging rebuke (Wasp-like) and no payment (reminiscent of the reactions of the poor to social assistance programs). The chronic form of such reaction is the undigested analysis.

At bottom, the whole complex often appears as an oral deficiency disease. Harlow's wire-monkey research could have been inspired by this kind of clinical phenomenon, if it wasn't in fact. It is as though they have been in training from earliest times to do without.

III

Sadistic depriving oral mothering experiences seem to be the beginning of the cycle. They give rise to: 1) overwhelming rage and a proclivity for primitive somatizing reactions; 2) premature self-object differentiation which yields inadequate self (empty) and object (no empathy) representations, aggressively and sadistically suffused; 3) a search for refusion with a good omnipotent object (religious hunger) plus the need for external enemies.

Wasp-a Protestant Disease, American Gothic, Or The State Of Waspishness.

Feelings of humiliation and simultaneous grandiosity equates to an identification with the figure of Jesus (an example of projective identification).

This maternal sadistic attack on the infant's neediness reflects her own mother's attack (subsequently incorporated) on her own emergent self, and represent a psychic form of child abuse. The subjects never achieve individuation, a healthy sense of self, or a unique identity (accounting for Roman numeral surnames) or maturation (remain children of God). In part, an attempt is made to overcome the lack of individuation within the institutionalized religion via sect formation. Schizmatic movements with a profusion of individual denominations takes place (along with a parallel process externally of social group formations, the "club" phenomenon).

There is an apparent overvaluation of "independence", not genuine individuation and autonomy but narcissistic separateness and self-sufficiency of an obvious defensive quality. What is being defended against is the feared/wished-for merging experience, which though longed-for threatens to annihilate the sense of self. In this regard, the conceptus in the womb must be viewed from the beginning as a malign object which must be pushed away as soon as possible, much like the adult love-object. (At present rates, the American population, overwhelmingly Protestant, is not even reproducing itself, a product of both effects above).

The defective sense of personal identity in combination with the reactive sense of superiority plus the felicitous (or consequent?) occurrence of English-speaking leadership in Western civilization in recent centuries combines to produce an avid interest and pride in geneology, whether personal, or even better, unblushingly in identification with leaders of Western civilization in general (The Mayflower phenomenon).

There is a susceptibility to intense envy of persons of other religions who seem more alive or who seem to have more (particularly Jews and Catholics), which leads to compensatory devaluation, attacks, intolerance, religious persecution, and reaction-formation with feelings of superiority and active proselytizing.

Wasp-a Protestant Disease, American Gothic, Or The State Of Waspishness.

The predominant warded-off instinctual expressions are rage and oral impulses regressively; depression, love and integration progressively. The rage and hostility (tonic-bound form) has been already touched upon. The orality (and the defenses against it) returns in our culture in a striking breast consciousness, disappearance of the practice of nursing (but not eating in bed), faddism...especially of food, drugs, and topical ideas, addictions (including work and religion), smoking, obesity and dieting, conspicuous overconsumption and materialism, a superficial optimism and outgoingness (manifested by the clubman phenomenon and "Babbittry"), and a deeper tendency toward dour pessimism and end-of-the-world phantasies.

The instinctual controls are rigid, spastic, inelastic, and ineffective (in the 60's known as "uptight"), the tension from which is so high (reflected in insomnia, muscular hypertonus and joint disease) that it demands relief (abuse of tranquillizers, alcohol, and the seeking of faddist relaxing methods and practicing of ceremonial releases), and often experiences spontaneous breakthroughs in the form of instinctual explosion (orgies of violence in our culture, mass murder in formerly well-behaved people, or group aggressive campaigns such as witch hunts within or wars without). The "sublimated" form of aggression emerges in the literary genre of the English murder mystery and the American fascination with mobsters and detective stories. The paranoid feeling of the enemy within, originally incorporated from the mother, becomes reprojected and provocatively induces in objects the hostility they fear in themselves (?American foreign aggression and domestic social unrest?).

The internal experiencing of aggression and non-satisfaction and nonexistence constantly samples death, which is rationalized as a virtue in preparation for eternity, which is compensated for by the fantasy of an afterlife with achievement of perfection and constant bliss. The poverty of affective and phantasy innerlife and dreaming is in part filled with incorporated recited religious dogma, slogans, and shared universal fantasies (commercially prepared sentiments, creating a market for the greeting-card industry).

The splitting and repressive mechanisms result in a lack of inner integration of the various structures resulting in inner disharmony, ineffectiveness, frustration and a sense of cross-purposes; hypocrisy, falseness, lying, acting, as-if phenomena, posing, double-life phenomena, and a spastic uncoordination; secrecy, witholding, stealing and cheating (corporate morality) are not at all rare.

The inner splits are also reflected externally, again, in a tendency to schism formation in the religion with a remarkable profusion of variant denominations. Equally notable is the toleration of this fragmentation, which can be valued oppositely depending on whether viewed as a pathological derivative or a social/moral asset. These same tendencies may also be reflected in our political organization of separate states and their ineffectual counterbalancing representatives, as well as a diversity of struggling unintegrated pressure groups.

The predominant fear is of disintegration, in such a poorly integrated state, always threatened by loss of control, of going crazy, which, if the defensive organization were not so rigidly stable (borderline, narcissistic character), would be a very real possibility. The predominant psychosis should be schizophrenic (and is in the U.S., once occupying 50% of all hospital beds in the nation), the predominant adjustment schizoid, with prominent hostile, paranoid features.

The primitive sadistic and depriving maternal imago becomes in time incorporated into a superego which compels the self foregoing experiencing need-satisfaction or pleasure (asceticism, martyrdom, Greek and American Indian philosophy), masochistic submission to authority, pleading for love through unworthiness, and a well-rationalized fatalism and modesty of achievement ("The meek shall inherit the earth.").

Later level guilt over the self-sacrifice of the idealized ancestors (son of God and Christian martyrs) compounds the inability to enjoy. An ego-ideal of achieving perfection through reunion with a suffering omnipotent God (religious ecstasy, also achievement of superhuman Godliness) completes the picture of the ego superstructures. The combination of self-denial and the fantasy of achieving Godliness equals the altruistic form of narcissistic character disorder which equals saintliness. Dynamically, the desire for perfection and self-abnegation is to placate the hostile object: Christian submission.

Superimposed on the earliest ego deformations are layered levels of neurotic formations: phobic, against contact; inhibition, of intellectual, affective and drive discharge (poverty of fantasy life); obsessive-compulsive ritualized drive discharge; guilt reactions from a severe super-ego; shame reactions from unfulfilled ideals of perfection; as well as assorted idiosyncratic conflicts, inhibitions, lack of sublimations, and symptoms of anxiety, depression, and mistrust. Anal retentiveness and witholding and overcontrol only in part represent a reaction against explosive drive pressures; in significant measure they are merely a psychic corollary and resultant to antecedent oral deprivation (i.e.,such a patient will "produce" more when fed).

Individualism and the rebellion against constituted authority, those valued qualities of the Protestant Reformation, found a ready application in the New World's geographical and cultural isolation from the Mother church and Fatherland, as an adaptation to the harsh environment, distance from even the local authority, and the necessity to function autonomously. However, this valuable historical adaptation has become fixed even in the face of changed circumstance, to the extent that collaborative social and governmental functioning has become problematic.

However, a happy invention has arisen to reconcile the opposing needs for family and separateness: the corporation, which enables impersonal association. I don't know if it was invented here, but we certainly have raised the development and practice of it to the "n"th degree. To be an officer or sit on the board of directors of a corporation is possibly the apogee of American ambition and accomplishment, easily surpassing the role of scientist, educator, professional, legislator, athlete, or artist.

Their psychology is of the newspaper variety (literally, avidly followed in papers, radio, and TV): glib, faddist, superficial, sloganeering, and unmoving. The total picture is that of an individual who is apathetic, politically plastic, conforming, intimidated, sado-masochistic, enduring, war-like, non-thinking, anhedonic, paranoid and hostile, yet tolerant and charitable, proud, unostentatiously "superior", and "good-looking". The internal state of unintegration is reflected in the external condition of the polity which is also unintegrated, comprised of stratified classes of "in's" and "out's" which accommodate the disparate attitudes within: "inferiors" are easily tolerated because isolated from the subject's own class, colonization becomes a natural social order for the "superiors", tolerance is advocated in general as a social good, but strictly eschewed within the subject's own class, which gives rise to the existence of hypocrisy.

The symptom of the abuse of alcohol is highly overdetermined, at least reflecting: 1) an oral craving (drinking and feeding on a high-chair from the bar symbolizing both nursing and infantile table-feeding); 2) an internal emptiness and coldness seeking fuel which burns to yield a sense of warmth and life; 3) an activity to fill the void of loneliness and boredom; 4) an anesthesia for constant psychic pain; 5) an antidote for unhappy sobriety; 6) a comforting attachment not obtained in current relationships nor memories of past ones (the drink, the bottle, and the bar as transitional objects of Winnicott); 7) a consoling reaction to felt rejection from an unloving object; 8) an act of defiance and rebellion against rigid (felt as cold and rejecting) partner, parental and societal expectations; 9) an infliction of punishment and destruction on the self; 10) a solvent for a sadistic superego; 11) an attempt to relax vigilance, to stop thinking and remembering, and to sleep and achieve oceanic fusion experiences; 12) an attempt to relax overcontrolling and isolating mechanisms, to fuse disparate elements in order to relieve unbearable inner intra- and inter-systemic tension; 13) an exogenous non-nutriment lubricant for interpersonal functioning; 14) participating in a social event with others who drink; 15) an identification with a distant parent who probably also drank; as well as 16) possibly reflecting some as yet unknown genetic factor in some but by no means all cases, separate from the characterological and psychodynamic features. Any wonder it is so refractory to treat?

This constitutional factor can neither be ruled out nor proven, but obviously must be kept in mind. All of the patients in my series derive from north-western European stock, the "Anglo-Saxon" in WASP.

IV

The acronym WASP we may suspect is overdetermined also, a constant feature of symbols which endure. The imagery of the insect is immediately called to mind, with its colorful anonymity, colonization in individual cells, genetic enduringness, dangerousness at close quarters, and oral aggression...including simultaneous sucking of juices from the host before egg-laying or envenomization...all could be seen as relevant metaphors in symbolic language for the character traits being described.

Indeed, object-relations often crystallize into parasitic arrangements wherein the sick partner "sucks the juice" from the more alive partner while simultaneously discharging his poisonous feelings into him. (These patients may represent the soil in which the British school of Psa. took root and flourished.) Such marital and therapeutic partnerships are not at all uncommon, and may open the way to exploring the psychodynamics of intermarriage. Already one reciprocal motivation seems to have been clarified: the Protestant's attraction to the acceptable closeness and dependency in the Jew's family, the Jew's attraction to the acceptable freedom and independence in the Protestant's.

Though the Catholic patient shares certain religious beliefs with his Protestant (very distant) cousin, incorporated in a general way similarly into his ego-superstructures, there are striking differences ritualistically and psychologically between them having to do with the oral and narcissistic phases. My typical Catholic patient's early phases seem relatively undisturbed, in fact eating is a part of the sacrament, as is family life the center of the culture. Impulse control is to a much greater degree regulated by mastery of sphincter control consequent to a good oral experience and incorporation of the loving parent, and by guilt from super-ego pressures, provision for the relief of which is built into the religion (the ritual of confession), the whole yielding an accepting, loving, integrated, lively, and humane picture. Indeed, when the "lid is off" with Catholic young people in late adolescence, an energetic sexuality and easy capacity for object-relations emerges. Not so with these Protestant patients, whose instinctual life is to a much greater degree inhibited by earlier pre-guilt intra-systemic factors, yielding the opposite picture of a denying, hating, unintegrated, deadly, asexual, and non-creative inhuman person.

To put it in dynamic terms, the WASP patient is attacking the baby in himself, repeating what was actually experienced in infancy. This psychic operation is mirrored in, among other things, Revolutionary Period American portraiture (which had its antecedents in earlier English formal schools) where there is a striking inability to render pictures of children which look like children-instead they are pictured as miniature adults. Pari-passu, a frequently-voiced fear of parents is that of "spoiling" their children. Adult patients tend to treat their own emotions (i.e.,instincts) as betraying enemies which must be guarded against. This also leads to an overemphasis on logic, intellectualization, and an over-estimation of the value of rules and laws, and processes of ritualization (vs. spontaneity) generally (e.g. British queues). The victory over instinctual presentations yields not only a sense of rightness and pride, but excessively so, to righteousness and superiority and a need to locate inferiors and scapegoats in the environment (which, along with the repressed oral and anal aggression, accounts for the esteemed position of canine pets in the society), while at the same time the private shame over inevitable lapses gives rise to an acute sense of hypocrisy, which in turn is struggled with by denial, projection, or rationalization as "the human condition". Contrast the absence of this concept in either primitive or better integrated cultures.

The healthy interplay of instinctual and defensive forces in the "normal" gives rise to a growth and evolution in the human personality, with an inner sense of excitement and discovery about what the future will bring, for it is essentially unknown. In these patients, however, an opposite phenomenon is present, perhaps best illuminated by the Protestant concept of Predestination (again reminiscent of East Indian class society and reincarnation). This sense of "fatedness", along with the sense of righteousness which accompanies it, can lead not only to a dour personal fatalism and giving up, but to its opposites, the idea of rebirth, and a sense of mission, leadership, natural superiority, colonization and religious proselytizing, noblesse oblige and "the white man's burden". In this view, other religious and cultural groups are seen as moral inferiors, primitives, children who are in need of enlightenment and control (the scapegoat or repository of their own denied and projected baby).

Of course all religions repose their undiminished individual infantile narcissism into the group, and in setting themselves off from others attempt to delineate themselves, apparent in zealous Jews, Catholics, Moslems, Hindus, or anyone else for that matter. What may distinguish the Protestants from the others, however, is a lively and energetic conviction of righteousness, which has, along with an equally energetic aggressiveness, led to (and in turn reinforced) assuming dominant control in their societies and the attempts to do so in others (missionary-ism?, Yankee Imperialism?). The record of religious wars and religious persecutions has not been a pretty one down through the ages, on the part of all religions, however.

V

That Protestants have made gigantic, perhaps even pre-eminent contributions to the world's accumulation of knowledge, culture, progress and human riches is undeniable, and in no way contradicts the thesis of this paper. Aside from the obvious "out" of distinguishing my patients from world class leaders, the fact that some achieve and some don't with similar character traits means that we are not yet at the point where we can evaluate the sum total of a personality from a description of his character, or, alternatively, a given structure can have exactly opposite effects in two manifest personalities. Also, to be remembered again, there were many Protestant patients I have had who did not correspond to the description given above, and I do not really know why; I expect, however, the answer to be found in the quality of their mothering, in turn from the healthier experiences with her mother.

As a society, I find the Protestant one to be fair and tolerant, almost to a fault, being unwilling to openly discriminate against some of its most destructive elements, to protect and preserve itself from outside and even internal attack. It is a virtue, this Christian charity and acceptance, but when carried to excess becomes a liability. Whether the attacks on the society mirror the internal state of affairs and are thus less noticeable, whether the magnanimity required of the superior host and its guilt requires overlooking them, whether coming to grips with the risks entails too much weakening of the defense of denial, whatever the combination may be, I simultaneously admire, am grateful to, and salute the tolerant Protestant society which harbors me, and worry for its self-destruction.

VI
May 29, 1991
A Psychoanalyst Looks at Alcoholics Anonymous (Addendum)

I have recently had the opportunity to study a so-called chemical dependency in-patient unit (so named in the East, more often and more accurately substance abuse in the West), run along the lines of AA by a team of mental health workers of mixed backgrounds led by alcohol counselors (often recovered users themselves), with the nominal inclusion of a psychiatric member for necessary codifying and prescribing functions, but more for legitimizing and marketing purposes than genuine collaboration, I fear. The experience was illuminating in several respects, particularly related to the themes in this paper.

First of all, the patient population was almost exclusively Catholic, predominantly Irish, some Italian, with rare Protestant and Jewish patients. The composition of the staff was unknown to me, but seemed consistent with the indigenous general population of friendly but moralistic, parsimonious New England Yankees. The philosophy of the program administered, directly drawn from AA, was nominally non-sectarian religious with overtones of both Christian divisions: an undisguised authoritarianism ("We know best", "You will do this now"), and a similarly undisguised public Evangelism with group confessions of having fallen, guilt, and personal powerlessness (and thus responsibility-lessness, and thus demonization of the liquor "bug"), an appeal to the Lord for help, an appeal to the group for support, and a process of purification which bordered on exorcism of the inhabiting devil...all covered over with a pseudo-scientific patina of "disease", which the medical profession, I fear, has too readily uncritically bought into.

Although there is a superficially open acceptance of anyone who desires to join the AA program, it is uncritical and anonymous (contained in the name of the organization and its practice: "No last names, please"). In addition and more importantly, the acceptance is highly conditional on identifying with the program, and thus experienced as partial at best. Along with the various strictures and prohibitions placed upon the individual, he would not be too far off to experience the acceptance as actual rejection with a thin gloss of "treatment" ("for your own good").

And actually, this is what the vast majority of the patients experienced in their home environment, being overtly thrown out of their homes for substance abuse, after having been covertly rejected out of, I believe, a cold nature in their partners or a parallel dependency there which likewise limited the support they were able to give. This seemed to be the most frequent theme in the histories. Many of the patients described spouses who seemed unable to love, too needy themselves, narcissistically self-involved, or described as "saints" (for their patient enduring of the patient's mis-behavior) while the patient readily accepted the total blame for their own "sinning" . Most of the patients came to treatment in the midst of physical separation, divorce, or court-ordered injunctions to stay away from the family. These patients (and not a few of their separated spouses!) were pathetically eager for a warm and accepting therapeutic relationship with a psychiatrist and worked very well and rapidly in it, demonstrating thereby a high degree of psychological-mindedness, insight, and capacity for object-relations as well as their deprivation of it. However, this good relationship was perceived by the staff as antithetical to the purposes of the program (as was any socialization or fraternization of the patients with each other) and was either covertly sabotaged or overtly countermanded.

Second in frequency was the theme of quite conscious identification by the men with their (dead) father's drinking (and their shared rejection by the mother), often down to the pattern of the drinking, behavior while intoxicated, and even the brand of liquor consumed; the women complained of un-loving husbands, displaced from earlier histories with their mothers. Next in frequency was the theme of intervention of the authorities because of criminal behavior while under the influence or in dealing narcotics (acting "bad"), with it's corresponding (?or causative) sense of guilt and ready acceptance of the punitive environment (to be sure, less so than jail time, although a surprising number opted for the latter given the alternative of a "therapeutic" disposition).

Equally frequent was the history of physical and/or sexual abuse in childhood, but because of its recent media popularization and the consequent hypersensitivity to the possibility among the patient population and staff alike (who also express the clinical wisdom that this finding is frequent among substance abusers), its real frequency ought to be more carefully studied, as would befit all of these etiologic factors.

There was a smaller sub-group of patients, a residual category if you will, that did not seem to share the psychodynamic characteristics of the others, consisting of apparent "losers" or people with inadequate personalities who had turned to drugs and crime as part of their social mal-adaptation, and who did not seem influence-able by any rehabilitation efforts, becoming recurrent relapsers and upon whom repeated efforts seemed wasted (not to deter the business of rehabilitation, however).

The related observation was the high rate of relapse and recidivism in the total patient population, and the staff's and administration's apparent ready tolerance of it, rationalized as just an expected normal aspect of the "disease". I could not escape the impression that there was an unconscious encouragement of relapse, effected by undue shortening of the "therapeutic" experience (rationalized as economic necessity, which was belied by the multiplied cost of repeated treatments, which suggests in turn the possibility of a more venal motive), and the encouragement of a regressive dependent relationship with the authoritarian power structure of the organization, which dependence was merely endured and ultimately discouraged out of simple fatigue and in the name of weaning. (This in contradistinction to our psychiatric use of regression as a means to the re-educative goal of achievement of genuine autonomy.)

I came away from the experience frustrated by the blocking of my therapeutic efforts and clinical expertise, and angry by the rebuff experienced at the hands of denying "helpers", but reconfirmed in my conviction that alcoholism and drug abuse are oral deficiency syndromes, a product of an attempted relationship with a non-nurturing object, with the abuse a symptom only, a seductive habit to be sure, the so-called "physiological dependence" a factual but thin, non-operative factor (many users give up their "habits" readily and repeatedly when conditions change: e.g. soldiers' un-hooking from heroin post-Vietnam).

This is not to say that for a certain sub-population of alcoholics, the AA approach is not a pragmatic and semi-successful attempt to deal with an overwhelming public health problem in our society. But we must be careful not to over-generalize this acknowledgement into a prescription for all our patients, particularly intelligent, educated, and relationship-able ones who can be and are helped by psychotherapy and psychoanalysis much more enduringly every day of the week in our practices. And we should be careful about our scientific conceptualizations of this syndrome: that should remain pure.

Freud himself spoke of the necessity of alloying psychoanalysis in the treatment of problems of everyday life, and this institutional approach to this clinical syndrome may be just such an example. However, the ringing in of Psychiatry by AA in hospital units variously described as "Dual-Focus", "Dual-Diagnosis", and "Dual-Track" may be less a synergistic collaboration than an uncomplimentary exploitation of us.

Repeatedly during preparation, the fable of the Emperor's New Clothes came to mind, with the author either perceiving what others were not wishing to, or being the last to see what everyone else already knew. Probably all in this society know this material preconsciously, and it remains for the innocent someone to blurt it out. Also, the relief and indignation personally experienced in lifting off a sense of accusation and guilt carried as a non-Christian in this WASP society is matched only by the trepidation and guilt in laying it back on where it belongs. The process has brought home to me the emotional dilemma experienced by the various non-WASP minorities in our Western culture.

The Jewish analyst is, to be sure, subject to his own cultural bias and insularity, manifested in lumping together all non-Jews as Christians or Gentiles or Goyim. Striking, however, are the personality differences between Protestants and Catholics, and their amenability to treatment. In several important dimensions, Catholics seem more closely related to Jews.

Contrary to prevalent analytic opinion, I do not see Catholicism as anywhere near the contraindication to analytic candidacy that Protestantism represents (in the pathological form here described). Though I would not go so far as to assert P. is an absolute bar to analytic treatment or training as some do, I do think it may be a relative contraindication which requires very careful individual evaluation by someone who has worked through the egalitarian myth of universal treatability and trainability.

This, of course, provides another paradox, in that the Jewish physician represent a doubly-tabooed object, and the patient to have already broken with strong family traditions. On the other hand the seeming contre-temps may provide clues to the growing phenomenon of religious intermarriage.

Cf. Freud's (1927) Future of an Illusion.

Contrast the American fast-food phenomenon and the European and Asian sit-down family meals.

The apparent absence of esthetics in American culture is, of course, a commonplace. One Italian analyst said Americans touring her country were readily identifiable as the only ones to wear plaid trousers.

One Christian Scientist/Catholic scholar describes the historic early Anglo-Saxon tribal wars and later Protestant religious ones as destroying all cultural differences amongst the conquered peoples, rendering an homogenized, "bleached" effect, contemporaneously known as "whitebread". Is this the analogue and source of the American political philosophy of elision of cultural differences, the anti-discrimination value, the melting-pot idea?

He contrasts the Roman Catholic church as having and celebrating the different cultural stamp it enjoys in each separate culture in which it exists.

The quality of impulse control is reminiscent of conditions conducive to stuttering, but that symptom was not notable in my series except in affective and excretory form.

If the Puritans did not have Red men to protect against they would have had to invent them, which indeed they proceeded to do in Salem. The picture begins to emerge of the possibility of our founding fathers and the Puritan culture as being seriously disturbed dissidents in breaking away from the mother culture, possibly recapitulating the experiences of the leaders of the Protestant reformation before them.

One cannot help but be reminded of the famous newspaper family and their counter-culture rebellious daughter in the news recently, possibly a paradigm for the counter-culture movement in general in our midst, whose adherents, labeled love- or flower-children, correctly perceive the underlying sterility of contemporary American corporate society with its essentially anti-libidinal position.

See addendum "A Psychoanalyst Looks at AA", part VI.

In the patients' unconscious, however, snakes and other reptiles most often symbolize these dreaded qualities.

See note on "AA" again.

The obvious association here is to the practice of abortion, so prevalent in our and Northern European Protestant nations, so abhorrent to Catholic ones.

Again, see the addendum, particularly how the Protestant staff treats the lapsed Catholic alcoholics.

Although initially puzzled by this seeming contradiction to my private practice experience, admittedly in a different geographic and socio-economic population, I came to the apparent explanation (or rationalization) that to a significant extent the drinking in this group was largely cultural, but their members' entry into a punitive and unaccepting Waspish "therapeutic" milieu was indeed reflective of their individual psychological histories: i.e., their happier cultural group fellows might drink, to be sure, but not to the extent requiring institutional detoxification.

The consequence of an encounter with a narcissistic object, as described in my paper "Toward a Unifying Conception of Narcissism".

BOOBUS AMERICANUS II

William S. Horowitz, M.D.
April 29, 2010

One of the highest ego functions of the human brain is the ability to discriminate, to detect the difference between two closely located stimuli, to be able to tell two from one. This can be accurately demonstrated and measured in any of the various modalities, e.g. two close points of light, two adjacent sounds, to near touches on the skin at various surfaces of the body, and so on. It even can be inferred in a higher ego function, the use of language, in the ability to tell the difference between two closely related synonyms, by nuance. Or in the case of a yet higher language function, the ability to detect the tone of a communication, the unspoken but inferred intent of the writer or speaker, the absence of which renders the subject tone-deaf.

This brief excursion into the realm of sensitivities illustrates that the human nervous system and its higher functions are exquisitely fine-tuned to the surrounding sensorium to which it is adapted to react. Thus the noun discrimination connotes a positive, nay a laudable capacity to exercise the best of human psychology. Even in the strictly scientific arena, the function of discrimination carries an indifferent neutral sense. It is only in the limited political sense that the word has a negative value...indeed, morally and even legally taboo.

One would expect to find that this ability is distributed in the population in a typical bell curve, with sharp and dull at the extremes, in the first two senses above. But, the striking finding is exactly that this ability is NOT smoothly distributed but heavily skewed in one direction, betraying the obvious non-physiological but highly politicized non-exercise of the function of discrimination. To be clear, a valuable mental function has been deprecated and forbidden for social purposes to achieve the dubious achievement of "social justice", resulting in the "dumbing down" of the American population at large. It constitutes a serious, nay grave handicapping of our society's capacity to function in the real world.

How is it that it takes a virtual lifetime to re-discover the simple verities that common sense had dictated all along? I have in mind here the realization that men and women are different, for instance; the realization that every married couple comes to appreciate in time, but that every pre-married couple blithely ignores as irrelevant. Or that adopted children from a foreign culture are different from homegrown ones. Or that the distinctive human races are NOT THE SAME as each other. And on and on.

It would be one thing, and an admirable thing at that, if our society were demonstrating acceptance instead of rejection of difference, toleration, a social and charitable outreach, an understanding, and a moral virtue. But that is not the problem, that is not the situation, in actual fact the ability to differentiate is inhibited to absent in the American public. By political credo, yes, by prideful rejection of foreign society's classifications and stratifications, yes, by guilt over the "unfairness" of difference, but from the outset by educational indoctrination from the earliest school years starting in kindergarten, where each child is given the shared task to clean the erasers. The "troops" are homogenized and conformed, the easier to deal with them.

How else do you account for a highly intelligent cohort of our society, the medical establishment, conducting disease and treatment studies for decades exclusively on males, then generalizing to all genders, and only latterly recognizing that female studies are required to understand the disease in the female? How else do you understand our national effort to expend human lives and countless treasure to "democratize" foreign cultures still practicing seventh-century mores? How else do you understand a Hollywood starlet unable to maintain a marriage adopting a "cute" brown baby to raise? I say they, we, don't know the difference...but we will.

POSTSCRIPT: News item April 30, 2010: Eli Broad is quoted as saying the Americans are rated 21st among nations of the world in educational achievement, being "Fat, dumb, and happy".

CITIZENSHIP-GULLIVER IN IRAQ

Stimulated by the national discussion being pursued by the president, Congress and the media, we, some of the people, are puzzled by the absence of creative options for solving the Iraq dilemma, It looks like "group think" is being advanced once again.

Why has not consideration of our country's past history been seriously considered? Have we not dealt before with indigenous, unassimilated, and/or conquered populations that have impacted our national interest?

Of course we have, utilizing the Possession or Protectorate or Purchase or Territorial political device to over time ease them into our political system. In the case of Germany and Japan we outright governed them while fashioning the institutions which would enable autonomous democratic self-government. The aim was either to incorporate the populations into our own, or protect our own from the militancy of the other. In both cases, the necessity of protecting and guiding the subjects whilst they learned the habits of self-government was shamelessly recognized and embodied in the policy.

One could analogize the maturing of a society to the case of the child who needs supervision while "growing up" to take on the obligations of adulthood. In our society, we allow 16, 18, or 21 years for the development of the capacity to become a responsible member of society...in earlier societies, this process was shorter, but in none was it ever instantaneous.

How is it that we expected the freed slaves, "3/5 whole men", to become full citizens overnight? Needless to say, it has taken them perhaps 100-150 years to become and feel full citizenship, not even the handful we allow our own children. How then do we expect the Iraqi population to assume the responsibilities of autonomous citizenry weeks or months after the elimination of their governor?

Could it be that our thinking is idealized when it comes to the issue of political rights? Are we under the sway of the revered principles of Equality and Independence so that we confuse them with measures of maturation? Does the infant have citizenship? In the sense of being born here, he is given the protection of the state; in the sense of being a responsible and contributing member of the polity, of course not.

One problem with this kind of flawed thinking is that it is irrational and unrealistic; it is, to coin a phrase, nuts. But in another sense, this mistaken thinking is moralistic, nay, messianic, and arouses the overtones of historical conflicts between our Western society and the Middle East, known as "The Crusades". It is highly provocative, to say the least, to societies which don't believe in Individualism, but rather Paternalism (Tribalism), which is what we are dealing with here.

Why don't we simply take over the country of Iraq as our protectorate, govern it ourselves whilst setting up the institutions for eventual self-government as that becomes possible, share the natural resources FOUR ways with the 4 factions involved, and make a success out of this misadventure? We didn't go in there to institute democracy in a suffering population, but to protect ourselves from its militancy. The democracy, if it comes as it has in previous times, will be a welcome after-effect.

Is the problem that we will be seen as empire-builders? Perhaps that is a time-honored technique of dealing with undeveloped societies. And anyway, we already are. Will be then seen as aggressors? We already are. Will we be seen as occupiers. We already are. Will we be unwelcome in the area of the globe out-of-bounds to us? By whom was this written? Why can't we unbound ourselves, using all our strength and experience to help ourselves and them in the process? Is there a conflict with our Western values? As UBL might say, they actually prefer the strong horse.

COMPETITION II

January 15th, 2011

DEDICATED TO THE MEMORY OF ROB MEYER

Where to begin? The manifestations are almost ubiquitous in human relationships, making a start or focus difficult. It can be found operative between teachers and pupils, those that offer, and those that resist, learning. It entails a generalized resistance to taking in. The problematic psychotherapeutic situation is emblematic of this resistance.

Where did we first encounter it? In the case of A.D.D., where the typical proband is self-taught, an autodidact so to speak. Such children, so numerous these days, are characteristically poor learners, for they do not fit comfortably into the usual classroom situation making disruptions to the disciplined process, often out of boredom. However, if placed under the nose of the teacher and paid focused attention, they seem able to function better. Or, alternatively, if they are left alone to satisfy their curiosity by themselves !!

It is true that they are benefited by chemical stimulants which have the paradoxical effect of slowing them down and functioning normally. What does this suggest? Another emblematic trait of these children: high intelligence. Putting these two together raises the possibility we are seeing a disparity between the child's capacity for learning and the teacher's lesser ability to teach (or a competition of the pupil toward the teacher). Did this typical child learn early on to mistrust his mother's offerings, and prefer to feed himself? I have found this history not rarely in my series of cases.

In my clinical practice in many different venues, a grouping of cases seems to form: a high incidence of A.D.D. in general, with the boys accepting medication and raving about its normalizing effects, whilst many of the girls were the exact opposite, refusing to be medicated, and refusing interpretations which promised to resolve conflicts. In addition they showed other forms of resistance, often manifested by attempting control of the therapeutic situation through seductiveness.

What does all this have to do with competitiveness? I think it does. I played competitive sports in school and succeeded easily at those skills I was good at, enjoying the game with other men, and never being particularly aware of their rivalry toward me – we had easy relationships. NOT SO with the girls, who were obviously vying with me as I assumed they were just like the boys and ignored it. What a mistake ! It is my naïveté, which perhaps other males share with me, which has totally ignored the problem. Is that male chauvinism? Perhaps.

Now that I am more aware, I see it in male-female relationships all over, patient-couples, relatives, and of course in the popular press. Of course Freud identified the rivalry in the little girl toward the boy a century ago. Perhaps recent social movements such as fem. lib. have exaggerated the phenomenon, but I think deeper developments have been more causal. I have in mind the accession of the woman into the workplace, the ease of divorce, the fatherless family, available government support, and the new social freedoms they enjoy. No longer do women really NEED a husband after being given a child, and I think they feel it even if not in awareness. Communicated to the man, it is a total wipeout of his essential function: to provide. He is left useless in the relationship. Likewise, he doesn't need, or want to need, someone who doesn't need him. There is no dependence, hence no partnering, only singleness – where both find their place.

Another obscured source of the problem is our American non-discriminating "classless society" where potential partners in true patriotic form ignore disparities between them which almost guarantee incompatibility. Racial, cultural, educational, intellectual, age, wealth, even physical differences of size can provoke strenuous rivalrous efforts in the inferior-feeling partner to prove him/her self "just as good as". This competition can render successful and accomplished men, for example, feeling completely ineffectual and impotized in their marriage. That, in turn, can lead

Competition II

to grotesque over-achieving and over-amassing of "goods" to both prove their heft and to deny neediness.

Is our society at fault? Can we go back? Silver and gold wedding anniversaries are becoming vanishing species; now they are debating other kinds of relationships between the sexes, or even individuals, as steps forward. We in the Western world are not even reproducing ourselves, as our Eastern rivals are gaining in ascendance. And we are counting on guns to save us? Ralph Peters has an usually perceptive analysis of human societies through the ages and observes segregation into like kinds has always been and still is the order of the day, not artificial political mixing.

DEMOGRAPHICS

William S. Horowitz, M.D.
May 13th, 2010

The Greeks had a word for it: demos = the crowd, people, the population; graphics = the picture of. This is a snapshot of the population of the Western (read Christian) world in the 21st century.

Various writers predict Europe's population will be majority Moslem by mid-century; likewise, America's will be majority Hispanic by then. White Christian civilization-producers for the previous four centuries at least are in decline.

How do they account for this? Politics are blamed for the European transformation: the development of policies of Socialism, or cradle-to-grave support of the people by the government in exchange for high tribute to them. The Economy is blamed for the American transformation, the shifting of its productive capability overseas in search of cheaper costs.

To some extent this is true, although it may be argued those causes are effects of deeper causes yet. What might these be? Well, for one, labor unions, at least in this country, originally organized to secure rights to work, have succeeded in their endless quest to render workers' lives easier, have succeeded in killing the golden goose. Detroit and the American auto industry have been rendered non-competitive and bankrupt; in a quite parallel development, the rest of American productivity has been weakened and much has been transferred overseas to eager workers.

Perhaps more significant is the effect of a century of wars which are still in progress, and which have decimated the young male population of Europe for sure and weakened ours. This has left in its wake a society of young and old, both ends of which require support from a productive middle of the society which increasingly cannot provide it, at least to the extent it used to. These young men were the strength of the society, the protectors, the workers, the inventors, and the procreators of the next generation. The influx of foreign people into these societies are filling that gap, but not in the mode of natives. It doesn't go unnoticed that we go about trying to save other troubled societies, and not unaccounted for, whilst weakening our own.

There are two pharmaceutical products which saturate the American TV screen with their endless repetition. One is to neutralize the effects of ageing on the human cardiovascular system and is the best seller in the whole industry, keeping it in fat profit. The other addresses the heretofore unmentioned inability to procreate children by impotent males...are they so numerous in our American society that they require this special attention? Apparently so, echoing the proposition above.

Which leads to the next possible factor in our demographic evolution. I have labeled our civilization Western in the style of many writers, but it stands in place of Christian, the predominant belief system in this part of the world. Does that belief system have an effect on the changes noted above? What about tolerance, of those different in our midst? What about charity to support the poor? What about bettering us and reaching for the good and ideal? Having faith in the betterment of mankind? Dispensing justice in confronting evil? Being compassionate and merciful? Exhibiting love, especially toward our enemies?

Do these laudable attributes render our society vulnerable, or invulnerable? Does their absence or opposite qualities render our societal adversaries vulnerable or invulnerable? One would do well to reflect that Jesus, the founder of the Christian faith, and his disciples were martyred for several hundred years, whilst his religious rival and antagonist, Mohammed, when he later arose preached making martyrs of his non-believers, the Christians he battled all over the old world. It would be a mistake to take this history, tradition, and expectation un-seriously.

DEPENDENCY

William S. Horowitz, M.D.
February 28, 2010

We humans are known for having the longest period of dependency during development in the entire biological kingdom, reaching our final adult form some 20 years after birth. How then could this fact NOT be the unending legacy echoing in our psychological lives from then on?

The human is a animal, needing the company of other human creatures who form both a larger human society and smaller circumscribed *societies* in which to belong. He also is most likely to choose a life partner with whom to spend his years on earth, a society of *two* until it becomes augmented by new ones

These life-long social tendencies are the obvious effect of having been raised into adulthood in the company of others, and specifically for an intensive period the exclusive company of *one,* his mother. This earliest human relationship has profound and lasting effects, recognized but mocked by every psychotherapy patient to his listener. As self eveident as this relationship is to objective inspection, it is characterized not by its affirmation but by its denial, We humans negate the importance of our early need for a mother, carried to an extreme by the so-called *Infantile Amnesia,* total forgetting of the first five years of life ! The process originates sometime around the age of two as the strengthening toddler begins to feels his independent capacities and first says "NO" to her.

But as this very. strengthening of autonomous capacities proceeds through development it falls into conflict with the earlier and still-needed reliance on the nurturer, resulting in the prototypical plea, "Please Mother, let me do it myself." with the implied, "But stand by me." Thus the human struggles his way to eventual adulthood, perhaps somewhat analogous to flying free of his familial cocoon when ready.

Dependency

This struggle toward independent existence in all spheres of that existence, physical, emotional, and economic, are experienced by the subject as his justifiable right of self-development whilst being resisted by others not so favorably disposed to him, his family (as though they would prefer to keep him helpless!) The "I" of "I need" becomes the "I who doesn't need, this or you!) And, Voila! We have before us the smug, self-satisfied, sarcastic, insufferable teenager whom we all are ready to be rid of. The preparations are complete!

It is this period of growing self-obsession that we therapists focus on. to the exclusion of his denial of his need for the *other*. Narcissism is the symptom of the withdrawal of interest in and need for others. It is a dynamic state achieved and maintained with great effort, the state of **Independence**. It is not to be mistaken for the successful culmination of a long struggle, an end-stage of development, but rather as a way-station on the road to mature adulthood, the productive interaction in the society of others, In short, socialization (or dependence on others); *that* is the achievement.

In our consumer culture this halfway house is manifested by amassing all the goods possible to pursue separate existence (as on a desert isle); in more reflective cultures, perhaps it would result in a retreat to a mountain top for contemplation. The greedy American is not portraying his skill at living well but rather displaying his negation of the need for others, the amassing of endless supplies, and the utter fear of being without.

We therapists participate in this denial, or delusion if you will, by focusing our attention on his self to the exclusion of his object relationships, which process is roundly enjoyed by our subject, the patient, reinforcing the very defense he is employing. So we note the "need" he, the actor, comedian, teenager, even political leader, has for so-called narcissistic supplies (attention and affection) in lieu of spotlighting what he is doing to his primary objects. **Here there is strong unresolved dependency, denied, manifested by strong angry attacks on her "inadequacies". This defense is originally directed at his mother, the re-edition at his wife when she becomes one, a too frequent source of infidelity and**

divorce. Without making him aware of this fact, we are colluding in his resistance.

But it is not just the therapist who can make this mistake, endlessly coping without results. You must have recognized that all of us in America place a high value on **independence,** in our history, in our people, and in our political relations with other nations. So much so that we have actively participated in innumerable wars of independence around the globe which have characterized the twentieth century. How much of this global movement may have been inspired, stimulated, and reinforced by us is worth pondering, as are the questions as to what extent we took one or the other side of the conflict.

This pattern is undoubtedly one important source of the charge of **"arrogance"** levelled against us. Are we the adolescent country just entering our adulthood, not usually acknowledging our utter reliance on the good offices of our neighbors. How do we react to the realization of their impatience with us: by more attacks on their *failings*, often by making more war. So, perhaps that "self-evident" legacy of our biology has blossomed into a problematic aspect of both our individual psychology and our political sociology.

It is true that we have come to the defense of the mother country Europe twice and helped save her from destruction, as we have with others, but it is also true we have tried to rescue colonial powers losing their grip on their independence movements. Now we are left with over 100 military bases around with world, not having sacrificed any territory in the process but possibly on the way to losing our economic hegemony to the emergent nations. On the other hand, it could equally be said that the tables have been turned and now **WE** are the mother country having inspired those nations to *emerge and vie with us*. It resembles an optical illusion how this perspective can shift momentarily from one to the other hand. Perhaps it is inappropriate to apply individual psychological concepts to geo-political ones. But are there better routes to understanding history?

Dependency

Some 200 years later, are we still waging **Wars of Independence?** Are we ready for mature adulthood, socialization in the community of nations? Is your child ready to join you as a practicing adult? And are your immature idealistic "liberal" political attitudes from high school (*"we against them"*) ready for realistic seasoning and respect for the *other*?

DIAMOND IN THE ROUGH

William S. Horowitz, M.D.
September 5, 2010

In my clinical psychoanalytic experience now of some fifty plus years, it has been a rare exception that a patient has presented himself with a classic neurotic or psychotic syndrome of two-turns-of-the-century-old Vienna. Usually they had what we would classify in retrospect as personality or character disorders, coming for help with chief complaints they were unable to verbalize. They were unhappy, to be sure, most often ascribed to a troubled marriage, in turn a product of an "unsatisfactory" mate.

If there were any commonalities in the group, it would be this history of unsalutary marriage. But in longer perspective, it became apparent that they were mostly highly intelligent students in their respective fields who had few if any long-term friendships and had irregular occupational histories. In contrast, for the most part they found the treatment situation comfortable and were willing to undergo it and the relationship with the therapist both before and after. In fact, they formed a rather stable, durable, and rewarding one in contrast to those in their outside life.

What was their problem? Why were they loners, without friends, adjusting with difficulty to prolonged activities with a team or group, many unhappy in their own families? The understanding slowly emerges for this therapist, who didn't share these difficulties in his own life, that these patients had a problem in socialization. They seemed never to have had the rough edges of self-centered childhood rubbed smooth in subsequent adult relationships with others, learning to get along, to subsume themselves to the group. It brings to mind a now-past (?) practice of sending young girls to "finishing school" to learn how to sit and walk and observe the conventions of polite society; its as though these patients never went through this process during the rough-and-tumble of growing up.

It makes you think: why? Three general areas come to mind. 1) The modern family with few if any close siblings; 2) the schools' economic reduction in extra-curricular group activities: teams, music, publications; 3) the current ethos of the "Me" generation.

He is raised without the expectation of having to deal with others in a give-and-take, learning to suppress his difficult, stubborn and sassy affronts with cooperative moves. Begging to be elaborated: by you?

Focusing on the psychodynamics, as the technique is wont to do, is of academic interest, perhaps sometimes of therapeutic benefit, mostly of distractive value, perhaps entirely irrelevant in these cases, for the relationship with the therapist seems to have the actual therapeutic effect. What is that? Contact with an interested but non-judgmental person over time.

One of my old teachers, Dr. Maurice Levine of Cincinnati, held the view that "relationship therapy" is a legitimate and valuable modality of treatment. One of my more recent mentors, Dr. Ralph Greenson of Beverly Hills, espoused the significance of the real relationship, in contrast to that of the intellectual supplying of insight. Dr. Bruno Bettelheim of Chicago taught the school of the corrective emotional experience.

I am almost coming to the view that the emergent young science of psychoanalysis enthralled me and many of my generation of medical students in the 1940's, and perhaps oversold its utility as a therapeutic tool, gradually disappearing toward the end of its century, and *not* because our culture's demand for speed. A fellow candidate, Dr. Richard Edelman, confided his impression even during training in the 50's that we were being prepared to practice the arcane art of Venetian Glass Blowing.

DUTY

By William S. Horowitz, M.D.

The soil was unredressed grievances of the Civil War on its anniversary, and the concern and largess dominant America showed to its international foes and allies alike postwar, into which the Democrats planted the seed of domestic entitlement: civil rights. This grew to include all minorities, women, youth, and immigrants of all stripes, wiping away restrictive laws and practices in the workplace, home, and national borders which had stood for generations. In our already heterogeneous society, in our Protestant society which valued fair play, tolerance, and charity, it was unthinkable to do other than the "right thing".

These societal attitudes and values became incorporated into the national character and thence into the individual character, replacing the former notions of duty (obligations to others and the state) by entitlement. It also led to forsaken obligations: divorce and child abandonment; disinterest in military duty, citizen duty of participation and oversight, and voting; unlevied and uncollected taxes; and ready outspoken dissent during national crises. Also related is the un-felt obligation to one's own ego-ideal or ethical or religious impulse, resulting in decay of morality in general.

This weakening of the conscience, plus the leisure generated by the victory over the battle for survival, plus the release of raw instinct for full and immediate gratification, has led to license and overindulgence, seen in the economic movements of consumerism, overindebtedness and corporate cannibalism; societal aggression in general; overeating and an obese society; sensuality and sexual experimentation including normalization of aberrant practices; and proliferation of drug abuse. Our character has gone the way of our waistline: flabby and instinct-ridden.

The founding fathers, exemplars of the citizenry at that time, were heavily duty-oriented, as part of their Protestant ethic and the national crisis which revolution and re-organization generated. It was a much more homogeneous society, religious society, and hard-working society, intent on survival. Everybody worked, hard, and was in the same boat.

There was a common external enemy, the authority of the fatherland, which helped homogenize and consolidate the fledgling society. There were palpable external threats to survival, the harsh conditions, which further forged the young society into a strong collaborative entity. All this became incorporated into the character of the settlers, namely the strength of purpose, the drive to survive, and the felt obligation to each other, the nation. Added to this was the flush of victory in their endeavor, which lent the encouraging imprimatur of righteousness and idealism to their existence. These very qualities, however, can be traced forward to have ultimately resulted in some overextension of national purpose and capacity which now may threaten the society's continued existence.

THE EQUIVALENCE GAME

William S. Horowitz, M.D.
July 14th, 2010

We see it all over: "The Jews are just as bad as the Palestinians, and they are no better than Nazis; the Christians were historically just as bad as the Moslems; the Republicans are just as bad as the Democrats; there's nothing to choose between liberalism and conservatism; the previous administration was no better than this one, etc., etc., ad infinitum.

Melanie Phillips ascribes the emerging era of non-judgmentalism to a global retreat from religious and rational values. Judith Wallerstein describes the child of divorce's avoidance of choosing sides. Many liberals' "anything goes" philosophy arises from a claimed exemption from the onus of reality because of their adolescent moratorium from it. Horowitz writes of the intellectual inhibition caused by the political incorrectness of exercising discrimination; and what of the immigrants straddling two cultures with divided loyalties, etc., etc., ad infinitum.

The result of expressing such positions is an absence of any position at all, a no-opinion, an amorality, a non-judgment, a studied stupidity masquerading as a sophisticated tolerance. How is then one to proceed in evaluating situations and possible courses of action to take? One can't, and paralysis results. Is this the explanation of the *apparent* passive acceptance of an obvious nascent dictator emerging in a polity, or the orderly marching to oblivion afterwards?

There are situations in world political history which the ordinary citizen cannot truly evaluate the merit of either contending side...to be sure... but nothing prevents the cafe habituae from having his *opinion*. But there are many, perhaps most, who merely go along with the tide, and we call them "sheeple". Is this the truism that the political chauvinist knows and relies on to carry out his mission?

The *cognoscenti*, those in the know, those elite, educated, opinion-makers, are often victims of this malfunction and fail to provide the society the early warning and action to prevent negative potentialities, and, in fact, are often the facilitators of the very malevolence they fail to confront. Unhappily to observe, Jews have been in this position historically, in Russia, Germany, and now in America.

This blind spot is not merely of academic interest only, for it has lethal consequences both for the group and the society at large, obviously. It would not be unfair to call the passive people *cowards,* the activists downright *saboteurs.* Responsible citizens have a grown-up duty to make a judgment.

THE "EXPERIMENT" HAS FAILED

William S. Horowitz, M.D. Torrance, California

June 29, 2009

Time was when the "huddled masses" of Europe were drawn to this "new world" by the millions at the turn of the previous century. What drew them? Obviously, leaving a worse existence for a better one. There was room for hope, of improvement in their situation when the ideals of our Founding Fathers lit aspirations all over the globe. They called it a noble "experiment" in people governing themselves, a democracy they labeled it, heretofore only known to the ancient civilizations two millenniums ago.

These immigrants were an unusual bunch, savoring their original culture whilst simultaneously becoming super Americans in their hunger to identify with their new homeland. Their children, in turn, unlike the native American-born who took their nativity with pride but also for granted, the immigrant children became super patriots, in large part contributing the balance of power to their new country's victory over the old world in TWO world wars...to name just a few accomplishments.

Around two centuries into the new nation's history, signified by some historians as an expectable turning point ("when the masses have discovered they can vote the treasury into their own hands"), the complexion of the maturing society began to evidence some deterioration. Marriage and reproduction rates began to fall, church attendance likewise, civil unrest led to fractionation of the united polity into diverse groups, crime and incarceration rates climbed, drug use likewise, and corruption in the governing class became overt and tolerated.

Corruption, possibly, has always been with us, in individuals, small groups, some localities, and at some times...but it was the exception, not the rule. THAT seems to have changed. Now, every day we are assailed with the news of yet other transgressions and disappointments, not to mention

The "experiment" Has Failed

a progressive slide in cultural values leading to unbelievable circuses of mediocrity and worse. The higher values seem no longer to count.

Former patriots wondered with amazement and disillusionment the growing trends in their beloved country. How could their formerly reliable and esteemed civil servants be caught "with their pants down" in such numbers and profusion? How could the policing powers stand by and not only do nothing, but often participate in the wrongdoing? How to account for this evident loss of civic morality, and on such a grand scale?

WE, the witnesses to this confounding transformation, are experiencing, in addition to frustration, anger, anxiety, disappointment, and sadness...as well as the brand-new impulse to find a safe haven from our own country...we are experiencing disillusionment. It is a feeling of loss of idealism, of aspiration, of trust, of solid values, of belief in general, of comfort. What the miscreants have done to US, I believe, to disillusion us about them and the country, is what THEY may have experienced in their activity in the higher levels of society that led THEM to the disillusioning acts themselves. We may be feeling exactly what they were feeling that led them to abandon their principles (and we our beloved country).

So, corruption may be a social contagion. Are we really aware that our whole society, our way of life, is at ACTUAL risk? I don't think so, but IT IS. There are modern Tom Paines sounding the alarm in blogs and on TV, but I don't believe we the people really believe them...rather regarding them as "cranks" or "misfits". We are complacent from success, and that's what corruption breeds in.

Who can save our beloved country? WE, the PEOPLE...we formed it, we can save it, it's up to us, NOT our "elected representatives". But our efforts will be inchoate until we have a leader to follow. God help us he is not a dictator who offers to "change everything".

THE GESTURE

William S. Horowitz, M.D.
July 31St, 2010

What does the bride and groom do when wedded? What does the principal and graduate do? What does the President do with the child with outstretched arms? What does the mother do to the returning prodigal son? What do the young lovers do espying each other from a distance and approaching? What does the newborn infant and mother do? What does the little monkey, also by instinct, do?

They all embrace, they HUG, the universal inborn automatic primate centripetal reaction to the other. It may or may not be consummated with a kiss, a second-level apposition of intimacy, denoting and communicating yielding to the urge to merge. Thus we betray our underlying human history of having been one and the magnetism still extant in it.

We even have in our armamentarium the anti-hug, the middle-finger or forearm salute, the off-fending push, the rebuke, the barb, the needle, the provocative remark designed to make distance. And, gentlemen as we are, we have the polite intermediate greeting of the handshake, which also can be warm or cool; not too close, not too distant.

Whence cometh this array of human gestures toward each other? We take these for granted, so in-grained are they in our experience, but they didn't arise from nowhere, nicht wahr? Where did they come from? They are derived, I submit, from the earliest inter-human physical contact in all our experiences, from the mother-infant one we all went through.

Can they be understood as social developments over time as the individual matures and has different greeting intentions to express? Undoubtedly. But can they be understood in yet a different way, reflecting perhaps the nature or character of the original holding experience between different

The Gesture

kinds of mothers and different kinds of infants? Can these be of different degrees of warmth and coldness? Can different humans have different degrees of comfort with interpersonal distance? Sociologists have long noted the pattern in this dimension in different geographical (read temperature), social, and religious groups, and now we psychologists should add personality or temperament.

What a fine distinction we are drawing here, but what a consequential one for human life experience! It's importance cannot be overweighted. How many friendships or even marriages have foundered on such a disharmony between partners, how many individuals have been attracted or repelled by the comfort level in certain social, religious, or political groups? How many have even felt alienated from or belonging to the whole human race?

Just one more thing to ponder in the realm of discrimination of differences.

GREED

William S. Horowitz, M.D.
August 28th, 2008

Long recognized as one of the seven deadly sins by religious thinkers, as well as by Hollywood as an affliction of contemporary WallStreet and American society, greed is seldom confronted by we who undertake the analysis of the populace's malaise. It has become ego-SYNTONIC, to resurrect a phrase.

Time was that thrift, saving, waiting, and lay-away plans were the order of the economy; not so today, when instant satisfaction, buying on credit, borrowing especially for large purchases, and mounting debt characterizes both the personal and national balance sheet. THIS has become the norm, the former the antiquated and thus devalued. "If you've got it, why not?" And this norm has suddenly become the focus of attention with the looming financial catastrophe facing this profligate world. To think that the frightening prospects facing us are the result of innocent evolution of the economy from poverty to wealth is bad enough; to suspect that they are the intended effects of malevolent manipulation is horrendous...but a topic for another day.

How do we grow so insensitive to greed in our own lives? Greed could be defined as want beyond need, as exemplified by Imelda's thousands of pairs of shoes, or Liberace's hundreds of pianos. Are we all not familiar with children engorging themselves into retching; with capitalists ballooning themselves into bankruptcy? It is unfortunately commonplace and perhaps somewhat amusing, certainly socially acceptable.

How do we become so inured to the presence of greed? Are we born that way; is there original sin? Have we become too successful as a society? You take your choice of beliefs; I, for one, believe while the capacity is present in every one, the actuality is engendered. How? Four ways come to mind.

Greed can be enabled by a parent; a spouse; the ethos of a group, vocation, or nation; by all those who encourage excessive consumption. Such an enabler typically is self-centered and unconcerned with the individual needs of his or her charge, augmenting their own excellence by such actions. Do we know societies that want more and more? Of course we do: our own.

Greed can be inherited, a legacy form so to speak, in families with illustrious or famed forbears, who grant their heirs to feel entitled to more as their natural right.

Do we know someone like this? How about political dynasties?

And greed can be the product of envy, the observation that others have more than we do, and we want it, too. This is the hallmark of class warfare, producing millionaire basketball players who never graduated school.

And as above, greed can be induced by the society itself, with its incessant bombardment to BUY, BUY, BUY! This can be a deliberate retail-induced policy; a simple evolution over time of a society upwards with differential generational effects; and/or a darker profit-induced extension of buying power to benefit the creditors, those dispensers of the credit, the individual and the central banks.

Undoubtedly there may be other sources, but what is more significant is that which is not sufficiently ego-DYSTONIC, the ravages of unbridled greed on our lives and fortunes. This is the link of the essay: we may actually suffer losses as a result of reaching too high! Do we assume all reverses in our fortunes are always merely mistakes in judgment, luck or fate?

Sensing ENOUGH is the signal our personal permitted line has not been crossed.

How does this work? Well, there are natural limits to capacity, e.g., the stomach holding only so much. This also applies to the body's tolerance for alcohol, sugar, morphine and similar treats. But besides those obvious conditions (not so obvious to the greedy one), there is the workings of the mind, the childhood mind, that one which early on was confronted with some limits of some kind, if not the appropriate ones. Thus is embedded a primitive sense of wrongness or GUILT, operating silently and behind the scenes but unerringly undoing the excesses accumulated by wanting more. Make no mistake: we all have this censor, whether or not we go to church.

What is there to do about it? Obviously, DON'T be greedy. How? By listening to the preventative and corrective: ENOUGH.!

GREED II

William S. Horowitz, M.D.
August 30th, 2008

Stimulated by rich associations to the prior essay by friendly critics that ranged far afield, two areas are singled out for elaboration here: the internal and the external domains of the phenomenon. There are a surprisingly number of interesting topics arising from this nodal point yet to be explored.

What do we mean by internal domain? What is the inside situation which gives rise to greed in us? Many have suggested it is a sense of inner emptiness, unsatiated and unfulfilled, that stimulates the desire for more. This state of affairs, this excessive hunger, can be the product of depression in the intact individual, to be sure, but typically does the opposite, inducing anhedonia. It can be the result of chronic starvation of meaningful satisfactions; the end product of ennui or the lack of stimulation; but most significantly, the absence of abiding beliefs, values, accomplishments, or self-regard. We could say this latter source and remedy of it would be the proper bailiwick of the D.D., not the M.D. It would be essentially a spiritual problem, not a mental health one.

Then arises the question of the external domain: what outside us can lead to the unending quest for more. Can this sense of dissatisfaction be engendered by the society? Can the nation as a whole suffer from an insufficiency of good feeling? Is such a thing possible in our multiassembled and historically variegated citizenry? One cannot assess this directly, of course; the field is too big. But, look at other societies, older ones, more homogeneous ones and more thematically consistent ones. Do all the countries strive for increasingly more and more of things, of wealth, of influence among other nations? Do some appear, if not downright unprogressive, at least satisfied with themselves? Perhaps the Scandinavian nations present such a model.

Does the older society, tried and true, distilled over the centuries, purified, consistent, inward-looking, have a QUALITY which the young and still developing societies lack...a stability which is a counter-value to the restlessness and experimentation and expansion the still-emerging ones manifest and boastfully parade as progress. Could one sense in this comparison an environmental factor in the genesis of societal want? What draws the American tourist to the old country to savor and wish to duplicate here? Is it possible the MORE society is LESS?

If impoverishment of inner and outer satisfactions can be understood as one of the bases of overconsumption in a society such as ours, what can be done about it? Who wants it? I believe the people do, feeling driven to buy and enjoying it less in this "capitalist" society. It is in actuality a predator society feeding on the consumers, only rationalized and justified and camouflaged as a capitalist one. The "robber barons" of yore are still with us, only moreso, and the new ones don't even donate the charities back which used to somewhat ameliorate their rapacity. This is not to be understood as an argument for a different form of government, but rather a plea for the old values, good sense and moderation, to resume their rightful place in our lives and nation. Greed is a sin; they always told us so.

Perhaps there are grounds for hope that this healing is already underway: that exemplar of a past age of excess, like the powdered wig, is already slated for extinction: the SUV.

GROW UP, ALREADY

William S. Horowitz, M.D.

September 6, 2010

When we witness the exasperated adult losing patience with his recalcitrant child, does that exhortation reveal an implication of volition in doing that? Do children grow out of childishness, or do they relinquish it? "That is the question."

In "days of yore" the colonial-period artists painted children as small adults, striking to our modern eyes, looking primitive. But wait, maybe another unwitting revelation of the state of childhood back then....when every able-bodied member of the family pitched in to share burdens appropriate to their ability: the little ones can certainly carry water, pull weeds, sweep the floor, etc. We expected it of them, and voila!....they were able and proud to perform.

There was an actual bonus in performing as an adult, as being recognized as one of them, to the child. Surprising? Does not the contemporary child beg, "Please, Mother, let me do it myself". The modern adolescent drives like he simply can't wait to get to where he is going, which also includes exploring in the back seat for something. The urge is still there. What could have happened to it?

The easy answer is that in today's political and economic climate there is no incentive to standing on one's own feet, remaining regressed has been made too easy. True enough, that is the apparent explanation, but is it sufficient? How does it explain, e.g., the many exceptions of people and peoples not only being self-sufficient but reaching heretofore heights of achievement? What is missing in our exploration?

The infant in the crib discovers agency, his ability to bring his toes to his mouth. The toddler discovers self, his ability to stand alone. Both are

Grow Up, Already

wildly exciting and practiced repeatedly. The latency child discovers others, and friendships become all-important. The adolescent discovers the world out there and can't wait to leave the family and become a part of it. The urgent progression is forward, ever forward!

What could possibly throw the gears into reverse? Think about it. What comes to mind? Fear, overwhelming fear. Of what? Of loss of everything, of all these accomplishments and satisfactions, of annihilation, the end. Our colonial ancestor had "only" the savage with the hatchet to be wary about; today's young have to consider the snarling dervish with cutlass in his hand, or worse yet, the thermonuclear knapsack on his back.

Starting in 1945 we began to train our school children in drop-drills in anticipation of the dropping of THE BOMB. Have we totally ignored the effect on their expectations, and thus on their behavior? Were WE, as children, commanded to FACE IT? So, absent a potent motivation not to, the child grows out of his childhood naturally; only in fear does he seem to be reluctant to relinquish it.

No wonder going back seems not so bad, not being ready to relinquish what was. But what kind of life is it not going forward? Furthermore, the necessity for coming to grips with reality is ever more important, nay, essential to survival. We started out this exploration from the standpoint of the puzzled adult, only to arrive at feeling sympathetic to the child, only then to recognize the necessity of integrating the two. How can WE adults bring back to life our stalled children? No quick answer here: something we must all think about. The atomic scientists, including Einstein, in their secret laboratories warned of the terrible unintended consequences of the bomb: little did they know of the hidden penumbra it brought with it outside.

No intention here, however, of diminishing the importance of what lies between the ultimates. We still have an adult need to expect of them, and they have a need to give up their childish ways.

HELMETS

By William S. Horowitz, M.D.

Recent debate on motorcycle safety and undue accident/injury rates has centered on the mandation of wearing a helmet, and the conflicting arguments over whether it would actually decrease injury rates and infringe on personal rights. What seems to be missing from the debate, possibly from the lack of appropriate statistics, is whether this approach addresses the problem at all, or is merely an attempt to do something, anything, to reduce the hysteria.

Anxiety is produced in the populace by, among other things, the idea that everyone is at risk and helpless against a menace, which mounts anxiety to panic and leads to irrational "protections". "Statistics" which fail to discriminate between populations at risk are a prime source of this induced anxiety.

(Witness the recent implication that everyone is equally vulnerable to catching AIDS, an obvious attempt to disguise the real culprits and spread the responsibility as broadly as possible. Interestingly, the grasped-for solution to this panic is also a "thing", which hopefully will magically solve the problem: the condom. There is as much chance the condom will solve the AIDS epidemic, as wearing asafoetida around the neck warded off the great plague, or a cross the temptations of the devil. This object with magical powers of protection is called a talisman.)

It is my contention that helmets are a talisman and totally irrelevant to the accident/injury rate, serving only to distract the public and the riders as well, while pacifying the mothers. If statistics broken down for age were presented to the public, I believe they would show what most riders and parents know: that kids don't belong on high-powered treacherously difficult vehicles in the middle of traffic, and it is they who are being killed or paralyzed at an inordinate rate, not everybody who rides. (Experienced riders feel safer on a motorcycle, in contact with the environment, than driving an automobile, isolated from the surroundings by glass and sardine-can thin metal and blind spots, believe it or not.)

The latest in an almost daily litany of articles is about 3 teenagers traveling in excess of 70 m.p.h. and weaving between and around vehicles when one "lost control" and crashed, fatally of course; whether wearing a helmet, clean underwear, or carrying a rabbit's foot are all equally beside the point. This is a totally preventable loss of young life, going on partly because of ignorance, partly apathy, and perhaps partly antagonism by the driving public which is understandably fed up with such recklessness on the highways (some of which public will actively pursue and attempt to finish off bikers personally, again believe it or not).

The helmet has actual protective value, sometimes, at low speeds and relatively low impact velocities, from cement abrasion as skin, hand and foot covering has for the rest of the body; in addition, it may provide some shock absorbing to the cranium, but that doesn't do much for the soft contents within. However, the trade-off here is reduced wind and sound contact with the environment, which can function to impair reaction time, and with young men especially give them a false sense of protection, both effects working to actually increase, not decrease, the hazard of riding. (Try driving to the glass repair shop next time your windshield is missing at 70 m.p.h.)

At high speed and high impact velocity, the helmet accomplishes nothing except perhaps keeping the ears warm in cold weather and saving corneas for transplant. The reason for this is clear if you think about it: a human in a high-speed accident becomes an air-borne projectile which on impact snaps the neck like a pigeon's. The helmet is not even there in the critical area, and by its weight and cutting edge may even aggravate neck injury. Imagine a high-diver fully helmeted swan-diving into an empty pool...that is what it accomplishes for the bike rider.

Helmets

The helmet is a shibboleth, a cliche, a pacifier, a dangerous myth, which almost all experienced riders (safe riders, by definition) ultimately discard, soon after their training wheels, if not prevented by regulation. The helmet is beside the point, focus on which prevents a public debate on the real issue: whether young drivers should be given the privilege of driving difficult powerful vehicles amidst traffic they are just learning to negotiate. (It is entirely analogous to the ongoing debate over condoms for the control of the AIDS epidemic. It is as though the attempt is made to find a way to get around what is patently dangerous and life-threatening by gimmickry, so the awful word "NO" can be avoided.)

We have recently seen that motorcycle manufacturers can be influenced and controlled by our federal government for economic reasons; why not for the preservation of the lives of our young men? What business do manufacturers have putting out vehicles which cruise at 110 m.p.h., top speed in excess of 160 m.p.h., for the streets and highways of this country? Why does our state government license them for street use? Why does California, which assesses vision, knowledge of laws, and demonstrated capacity to control a vehicle at low speed, grant two-wheel driving privileges to young people who by definition lack the experience, driving judgment, and ability to handle themselves at high speed, and without so much as testing whether they can? Is this some sort of distorted civil obligation? Are all old folks who can't see or hear or move with alacrity also automatically accorded the privilege by policy of driving the freeways?

Why do insurance companies insure such vehicles for use by young drivers? Why do parents buy such vehicles? For the young person who is interested in thrills and trying his skill, it is as though his whole society quietly assents to his breaking his neck, without a whisper of reservation. THIS conspiracy of silence, against young men, is what this letter is all about, and which I plead with you to break. Say NO to motorcycles (and a few other things) for kids. That will cure the problem.

What, then, do I advocate? The age of 25 and a certificate of completion of the Sheriff's motorcycle safety training course for new licensees, the latter for renewal of presently licensed bikers between 15 1/2 and 25. And, the banning of racing vehicles for off-trackstreet driving, exactly as with cars.

The rhinoceros, the Sherman tank of the animal world, has relatively poor eyesight and hearing, but, then, on the other hand, he doesn't really need them. Muzzle the head of an antelope, covering his only protection, his sensory organs, and you cruelly consign him to certain death.

HOLIDAZE

December 23rd, 2010

Most adults, when speaking frankly, say they do not enjoy the interruption in their daily lives occasioned by a holiday, particularly a protracted one. They experience it as disorienting, boring, somewhat frightening, sometimes accompanied by an "end of the world" dread. Only the children look forward to the holidays, which promise a break from their school duties and the expectation of gifts. But even they give in to the boredom of random activity, leading their tired mothers to find something to occupy them.

Why this negative reaction? Not surprisingly, we punish a misbehaving child by a "time out", sending him to his room alone. We mete out the penultimate punishment to a prisoner by solitary confinement. The underlying principle seems to be that the social animal called human doesn't like being separated from his familiar world, the people he lives with daily. (It is only a surcease or relief to the rare individual we call a "loner".)

How did the holiday come about? It is usually rationalized as a celebration, at a time in the annual cycle of the society's life when natural, or supernatural, events gave reason to take a break from the daily toil of existence to rest and to give thanks to "the powers that be". The harvest would be such a prototypical event. The mystics, who have always been with us, succeeded by the clerics of organized religion, succeeded in turn by the politicians, finally by the retailers, have found these occasions as ready-made useful excuses to champion their own particular causes by co-opting them as celebrations of their own. The holiday, or break from routine, is the thing, not the particular coloration it has assumed.

What, then, is the function of the holiday break in human society; the "time-out" we have become tortured by its overuse? To understand it, we must realize it has diametrically opposite effects. As noted above, it isolates an individual from his daily confreres, but it simultaneously brings the mass of isolated individuals together in some sort of observance, a "mass" the Church calls it. Could it be that the ordinary citizen is perfectly willing to exercise his freedom to go his own way with whomever he chooses, which by itself would function to disperse the polity to nothingness (an effect of the "expanding universe?), but that this eventuality is a powerful incentive for the various levels of power-seekers in the society to exercise their wish to cohere or gather together their "flock" under their control? And maybe it isn't just an occasional rite we are discussing, but one utilized monthly, weekly, daily, and even many times a day.

Is this sheep and herder analogy offensive to you? What are the chances of a de-celebrating, de-ritualizing movement succeeding? We are in their thrall, those who want to control our existence, and it is why we fight for our "freedom". Are their genuine causes for celebration in our society, or to observe something as a whole? Indeed yes, more precious in rarity....as is anything else.

INTEGRATION

William S. Horowitz, M.D.
June 27, 2010

These essays have been an attempt to present a unique perspective on the human condition, to achieve a vertical integration among the various fields of study. They include here the realms of mythology, history, biology, evolution, physiology, psychology, sociology, and politics.

To launch directly into one of these perspectives, the Jews 2000 years ago broke with the then-tradition to introduce a novel idea which marked an inflection point in the march of human "progress". They replaced the then-concept of pantheism with theirs of monotheism, which has held sway throughout the ensuing history, even spawning divers derivatives of it amongst non-Jews. This was an event of permanent significance in human history, and could be characterized as a Declaration of Independence from what had gone before.

Far from universal credit being rewarded by the rest of society, Jews have been the targets of unremitting calumny for these past 2000 years, in varying waves of intensity, today marking a recent rebirth. Why? How to understand?

In the maturation of the human being, we have seen a gradual preparation during adolescence for cleaving from the cocoon family to a state of separate existence. The teen-ager develops a disdain for his former loved ones, a contempt, an assertion of non-need, an adoption of strange and unique habits of living, in general an estrangement from all that held him before in thrall in order to break that bond.

This declaration of difference arouses in the family an equally powerful readiness to be done with him, and "the sooner the better !". So, there is

Integration

general agreement with all involved (except perhaps a tearful mother here and there) that the adolescent can go, and "good luck !".

Now, this is not the end of the story, obviously, for in short order he surveils his environment to find someone who wants him. And in short or long order, he establishes a new family of his very own. He is now in the process of undoing his separation, and rejoining the rest of society, re-integrating into it. And his original family and the rest of society rejoices in this normal outcome.

What's with the Jews? Simple. They are stuck in the declaration of independence, like it is the desired end-stage of life, and they hate and the rest of society returns the compliment. And it can be reliably predicted that it will remain this way until the end of time, or until Jews decide they are human just like the rest of us and rejoin us. But they steadfastly assert to their followers that the greatest threat the group faces is that of assimilation, which we can clearly see turns out to be the exact opposite: segregation. Can they remain distinctive, identifiable, their own kind? Of course they can, but not by asserting they are different.

How do they do it? Let us count the ways: their own idiosyncratic calendar not used by the rest of the whole world, their own unique day/night cycle, their own day of the Lord, their own alphabet antedating "modern" Roman times written backwards yet, their own language last spoken in biblical times, eating a diet prescribed by prehistoric standards, proudly parading on TV in 17th century Polish costumes, walking the American streets in black-hatted hirsute retro style, etc.,etc. How disdainful of the rest of us can they get?

The Amish and Mennonites in America resemble the Jews in their appearance and abnegation of contemporary living styles, but, interestingly, in both groups the young are leaving their elders' ways and integrating into the mainstream. There is thus hope.

Integration

In the 17th century, the American Negro slaves faced a similar contretemps, being forcibly imported into an alien society. Being different, they were rejected as "equals" and had to undergo at least 150 years of struggle post-Abolition to BE accepted, far from complete today. During this time the Negro society developed its own unique culture, for self-preservation to be sure, including language, values, habits, diet, and countless minutiae of detail. Maintaining their difference became self-preservative, they thought: "No Uncle Toms, no acting white".

But we see that the strict adherence to difference, the refusal to join the surrounding society, has served exactly the opposite function: to arouse suspicion, antipathy, contempt, and outright hatred. If you have experienced a well-spoken, intelligent and educated, successful Black citizen, you will recognize that the shibboleth of the "color of their skin" becomes irrelevant and is automatically overlooked in favor of relating to a kindred. So, the Negro perhaps has also fixated on his Independence and difference, his refusal to integrate with the rest of the society in which he now dwells voluntarily, arousing the very "prejudice" he complains of.

Come to think of it, we have a new subject to add to this hoary old problem: the Moslems, also firmly separate and differentiating themselves from the rest of humanity and declaring WAR on it. WE humans, some of us, assert our difference, while the rest of humanity finds that unacceptable. Some religions attempt to heal this problem by declaring the universality of mankind, but in the process aggravate that very problem by their sectarianism (difference).

Assertion of separateness is antipathetic to society and is adolescent. Recognition of being one with mankind is welcomed and mature.

INTIMACY

William S. Horowitz, M.D.
June 15, 2010

Intimacy = closeness = learned at the mother's breast = being as one.

We attempt to recapture that rapture in marriage, and for a time it succeeds...until a third one interposes...or how it seems to the man. The woman's intimacy continues on unabated with the new one, while the man vainly searches to recapture it somehow.

What is mischaracterized as "sexual" is the attempt to achieve this closeness with another; it is more an infantile emotional re-union than something more mature. It is also mischaracterized as "infidelity" or "cheating" by the moralists or self-ish ones, who want to capture and control the wanderer for their permanent own. But in fact, the strayer is paying silent tribute to his original union partners, his mother and his wife. Sad to say, too often this eventuality spells the end of the shared phantasy for both partners, laying the groundwork for single or multiple divorce and marriage, siring of illegitimate children, and possibly fulfilling the biological role of the man to re-populate the race. This can be carried out in civil society, to be sure, but over historical eons it has been carried out by conquering armies by wholesale rapine, resulting in a rich mixture of genetic traits in the various societies.

Is this path ironclad? Can these forces be overcome and the marriage preserved? Of course it can, our experience tells us, but we recognize preserved first marriages are fast becoming the exception rather than the rule, unlike our grandparents' era. What it requires is a shifting of the desired intimacy to the family rather than exclusively to the individual...which then may eventuate in the formation of a large family or even a dynasty of successive generations, for instance (which are not particularly known for their fidelity, paradoxically).

Intimacy

Can the achieved intimacy between mother and child persist over time? Of course it can, often resulting in "special" relationships between her and one or more of the family's children, or between sibs. And fathers can have their favorites, too. The varieties of possibilities are endless: perhaps the take-away is the realization that strict equality of relationships between family individuals is NOT the norm, estate lawyers' and sob-sisters' counseling notwithstanding. It is difficult to be intimate with many.

IT'S NOT FAIR!

William S. Horowitz, M.D.
October 4, 2010

Who amongst you has not heard this plaintive cry from your child? It is ubiquitous, and emblematic of the childish mind which recognizes in it's globalizing, idealistic, and needy state the irregularity and unevenness in this world....as well as his own disadvantaged condition. It has hence been recognized for it's powerful appeal to all the other weak members of society, and so adopted as the policy of the liberal like-minded leaders and their believers. Not so much adopted, actually, but empathetically agreed to by the similarly-oriented immature liberal philosophy.

Its beneficiaries, of course, enthusiastically endorse it but it is also grudgingly given in to by the not-so disadvantaged members of society who are vulnerable to the forces of guilt and tolerance. We call the resultant sociological contretemps class warfare, or, the struggle between the "haves" and "have-nots". It has been successfully waged all over Europe, where it is in the process of failing of its unreality, but is renewing its assault on the American society presently.

Rush Limbaugh has recently enunciated an analysis of the resultant world-wide economic crisis, which lists as it's primal cause the avowed and implemented plan by the Federal Government to universalize private home ownership.... to alleviate the manifest unfairness or disparity between the rich and the poor. This necessitated, by means of irresistible bribes and compulsions, the compelling of financial institutions to offer mortgages to those who could not afford them. Only then, secondarily, did the banks engage in their devious inventions to protect against a total loss to themselves, only relieving them of a portion of the responsibility for the crisis which ensued, but utterly failing to protect them from the loss in the long run. It could be speculated whether the liberals' aim was two-fold: to house the poor ("spread the wealth") and to break the banks.

Pundits are explaining, and complaining, all over the media their inability to understand and fathom the administrations' strategy, likening it to varieties of STATISM manifested through history all over the world. That is the name of the political arrangement, but that is not the reason. The dynamic which drives such a movement is a product of immaturity: the wish for perfection and an all-supplying parent. The fallacy of the wish is just that: it is a wish, not a REALITY. Liberals, like children, deal in wishes, are utterly unable to deal with the real world and always fail, disappointing those who entertain a HOPE that their or their father's DREAM will come true.

Growing old and growing up are not the same thing.

JUDGMENT

William S. Horowitz, M.D.
April 11, 2010

We think of judgment as one of the higher ego functions, possibly processed in the frontal lobes and vulnerable to organic damage. It is a complex function utilizing many sub-functions as will be seen. Although errors in this function are often (perhaps too often) ascribed to organic damage, there are dynamic factors at work that can also explain its mal-function.

The age of the subject, his experiential history or lack of it can be a factor; the speed of ego-functioning can affect it; interferences in his visual or auditory comprehension of his world likewise; pattern recognition may play a part; of course, memory loss would be an obvious causative agent; attention is obviously crucial; lastly, the super-ego evaluation of the consequences of an act (or lack of it) can be determinative.

To exercise judgment, one must imagine what one can anticipate in the future after an act (this now involving a time sense). Imagining involves an appreciation of what follows what, the linking of cause and effect. This involves an idea of the outside world, external to the self, and its qualities and likely forms of reaction.

Now we come to the possibly central factor, a normal appreciation of the other, rather than an exclusive focus on the self. Egocentricity and narcissism, in all their varieties can and undoubtedly do result in egregious neglect and assaults on the whole world which lies beyond one's own skin. (For some reason, politicians come immediately to mind.)

We train young people to take their time, to restrain their native haste, in order to exercise more reliable judgment...which provides the clue to better handling of all the sub-functions that go into that judgment, thus confirming the modifiability of that function.

TO THE LETTERS TO THE EDITOR:

February 25, 2006

With the foreboding events in the Middle East worrying us all, I am reluctantly coming to the conclusion we are following a flawed strategy in our war with Iraq which likely will lead to failure: to wit, to attempt to "unify" that country.

Having witnessed the instability following WWI & II's post-war attempts to make "nations" out of distinctive political entities, such as occurred in India, Yugoslavia, and Czechoslovakia and the ensuing disruptions when the ruling power left, one would think the lesson would have been learned that this British empire model doesn't work, certainly in the absence of an overwhelming naval power or ruthless dictator holding it together.

Are we left holding the British bag, the sun never setting on our armed forces around the globe? And are we "tone-deaf & dumb" to the obvious differences between the various tribal factions as we try to impose a forced marriage upon them?

What could account for this strange uncommon-sense behavior? Well, to set aside cultural scotomata for the moment, perhaps we do it because it is AGAINST THE LAW. Yes, we are not permitted to discriminate, for to do so is un-American. One of the highest thinking capacities by which intelligence is measured, the ability to tell one thing from another, discrimination, is tabooed in our roster of social values. To be dumb, naive, excessively tolerant is honest and praise-worthy, to detect the relevant fact in a background of information is sharp, suspicious and blame-worthy.

America rightfully can be lauded for its ideals, courage, and humanism, as distinguished from the tired morality of the old world, but being sophisticated is not all bad, nor is being practical. Does this remind you of the profiling argument, too?

William S. Horowitz, M.D.

MY PASSAGE

William S. Horowitz, M.D.
September 8, 2010

Thinking over my long career in psychoanalysis, and having come recently to the understanding that much of the therapeutic value of my treatments rested on the patient's relationship with me (in contrast to the classic shibboleths we were taught), my mind cast back three-quarters of a century to my original honeymoon with training. And well I remember the mighty struggle I experienced between my love of hands-on general practice, and my fascination with the "new Viennese science". This was so strong that I took a whole year off as a practicing G.P. before launching into the first step of a psychiatric residency.

Now, the older literature stressed the pivotal technical importance of maintaining the "blank screen", the better to identify the elements of transference cast upon it. Only on further reading did I discover that the master's own technique was short and often involved every-day activity with his patient in treatment, including walking and eating together. Only on reading Young-Bruehl's biography of Anna Freud with its detailed history of the whole movement did I come to realize the disparity between the followers (not founders) of the European profession being frequently women, lay-trained, and Jewish, in contrast with the Americans with their strict qualifications for membership (M.D.), technique, and "holier-than-thou" WASP-like purity, stringently weeding out "irregulars".

In retrospect, it appears as though the original Viennese sacher-torte was hi-jacked, idealized, crystallized, intellectualized, immunized, isolated, wrapped in plastic and marketed as American "new and improved". All the "juice" had been wrung out of it rendering it a proper scientific method in the eyes of the authorities. My patients, on the other hand, have something different to say: that my "humanity" made their treatment possible,

My Passage

in distinction from the technique. Where would you place Sigmund on this spectrum? As he was not embarrassed to make known, "Not in America".

To make up for the absence of specifics, and for those personally unfamiliar with the couch rendering the allusions failing to resonate, what I am saying is expressed simply, "Its not the words, its the music" that make it work. Is it any wonder, then, that following the founding fathers of the inner circle, the "first responders" were chiefly women, and Jewish?

What was the irresistible fascination to the young candidate-to-be? I well remember the appeal of the possibility of reconstruction, of restoring to ab initio, of starting over someone's life which had gone off-track. That potentiality, compared to merely fixing that which was mal-functioning, was the decisive winner.

When I wonder why that appeal, I can't help but think of my beloved mother's facial and breast injuries which dominated my childish cognitive thinking for years, convinced women must come in one of three varieties: one right, one left, or both breasts. But, the impact was even broader than that, since talk and evidence of illness and doctoring was rife in the family (father and sister, too, had chronic conditions), which I believe was a major determinant of my choosing medicine as a career altogether. I did not choose doctoring by heritage, relatively rare in the professional group, but by early assignment.

All right, here comes the traditional question: would I do it all over again? I rather doubt it, as O.B. has retained its second-place allure over the century. The problem with psychoanalysis is that you can neither reconstruct nor fix "it"...but never- the-less it has been a most rewarding professional life for me and most of my patients. However, business, American-style entrepreneurial business, has increasingly drawn my attention through the years: inventing or offering something in great demand. Is this Anna Freud's Altruistic Surrender?

ON ACHIEVING PERSONHOOD

William S. Horowitz, M.D.
20 September 2010

What is that? It is a stage in the ongoing process of maturation in which the individual discovers, perhaps for the very first time, who he is. It is self-discovery unlike any that may have preceded it: unlike the infant exploring his very own body, unlike seeing himself reflected in the eyes of his parent, unlike the adulations from his friends, unlike the graded performance from his teacher, and unlike the received rewards from his adult world.

The sages, through the ages, said, "Know thyself". But how? Self-knowledge is not easy, is not automatic, may never be achieved. We are not built to look inward. We have ideas in there, to be sure, sensations, emotions, perceptions...but we don't KNOW who we are...like perhaps either a lover or an enemy might instantly identify. They can see us; we can't.

So, how to accomplish this valuable insight, arrive at this precious state of being? It is done, I believe, through WRITING. When you sit down to express yourself, on paper, about what you know, you will reveal who you are...for all to see, including you. An almost magical transformation takes place, a crystallization of self-identity into a somebody, rendering you a unique individual. No one can grant you this; you must accomplish this for yourself...and when you do, you and everyone else will know you as a person.

Do not mock it, do not avoid it, this is a, perhaps, the most rewarding experience of self-knowledge possible. When we expose ourselves openly, it vanquishes finally the shame we all carry. You will then stand tall, proud and self-assured to walk amongst men and live your life as you choose.

When you know who you are.

PLAY

November 29th, 2010

Juveniles of all the biological species engage in random content- less behavior that we designate as play. We rationalize it as practicing what will become mature intentional acts (and indeed it may serve that function over time), but it may merely be discharges of inborn activity patterns without thought.

Playing is not confined to the juveniles, however, for it is ensconced in the language of adults: playing a scene, playing the market, playing house, playing games, playing around, etc. These connote acting something, non-serious behavior, pretending something instead of authentic real intentional activity. Thus, for the adult, play has either a recreational or a somewhat degraded value. It can either have a refreshing escape effect (recreational) from the realities of life, which Freud signified as only work and love (and we add ageing)...or it can have the effect of purposefully *evading* the rigors of the serious life and only *pretending* to be serious. It is the latter use that draws our attention.

Playing with oneself may be the "transitional" phenomenon between the infant's sucking its own toes (and later discovering the pleasurable activity of manipulating its genitals, now a definitely purposeful act), and relating to the other. Masturbation then is an originally self-directed intentional act, which can serve the function of bridging to a shared activity with another. Children can (and do) play with each other, and so can adults, arousing pleasure but not necessarily involving serious loving intentions... though it can be a part of the sexual foreplay that can lead to that aim.

Why is this important? Because *not all sexual activity is the same:* some is merely juvenile play, and the actors will confess (to their betrayed partners) that "the fling was meaningless and I don't know why I did it", and some is for real and serious "and I love only you". This is by now a near-universal story familiar to us all, but approaching in popularity and frequency these days is the occurrence of homosexual activity and its cognate, *playing house.*

Because it involves the participation of the sexual organs, we make the mistake of equating it with mature adult loving family building. It is not; it is only the *juvenile* form of the latter, passed through by *all* in the process of maturation, a sufficient dynamic in itself *not* necessarily requiring unique hormonal or genetic factors (which remain to be convincingly demonstrated). It is only that they, the homosexuals, never passed through, or maybe regressed to, this intermediate stage.

I remain impressed with the finding among my homosexual analysands that a typical history of strong infatuation with the mother, a literal love affair, existed before the age of 5. And I have also come to believe that this is absolutely typical of *all* boys. The implications are obvious.

POLY SCI 101

William S. Horowitz, M.D.
July 27, 2010

This is a lesson from the free (not for long) university of the Internet, for all those of you yearning for something free. It is a lesson in basic (that's ABC's to you) social formation under which people live, nowadays.

In the old days, there were cave families, hunter/gatherers (men and their captive women), village collections of those, then larger cities, then even larger states, then entire nations of states, then for the past several hundred years our present societies. The Church and its rules (dogma) were the prevailing force up to the so-called Enlightenment, when reason (individual logical intelligence) overthrew the collective mind-control prevailing around the 1500's.

Unsurprisingly, certain individuals and their families and their friends became dominant, often by virtue of "inherited right", and were called royalty. The sub-royals were given large tracts of land on which crops were grown by the commoners called peasants or serfs. This constituted the medieval society ("All for One"...or a few: Oligarchy).

Two hundred years later the French nation revolted against this arrangement, establishing the era of the "common man" or Republic, and following their example, the Americans split from their English parentage and became a Democratic Republic.

Since then serving this common man became the motivating force in the further development of both societies, but in very different ways.

All those who wanted to be taken care of, including the young, the aged, the ill, the poor, those wanting more, those disinclined to work, those feeling entitled, and those merely wanting to imitate their superiors and game the system, they all tended to accumulate in Europe, where they were seduced by the siren call of the collectivists who offered "everything" to the masses but actually took everything for themselves. They were known variously as statists, communists, fascists, or socialists. In less formal terms, they were kleptarchs or oligarchs. Who were these people? The old aristocracy, the money-bankers, the political dictators, and often members of a small immigrant exogamous group, uniformly enriching themselves and their Swiss vaults with the wealth of the nation.

All those attracted by the siren appeal of individualism were attracted to America, where they could breathe free and make their own way by their own efforts. This collection of individuals and attitudes and efforts built the most successful society ever seen on earth and was known as capitalism. But after a decent period of defending itself and most of the rest of the world through its strength and sense of fairness, the people who held the power in the society began again to hear the siren song of "unfairness and re-distribution" and faltered. (Can an entire society feel guilt?)

Now we are engaged in a perilous struggle between the old world ways (now turned new) and the new (now turned old), for which so many have valiantly given their last full measure of devotion. It will not be long remembered what is written here, but we will weep with deep regret if we dishonor our brave forerunners and forget their sacrifices that won the good we have here.

POME
AUGUST 12, 1995

When Nicholas was
a little boy,
he amused himself
with his little toy.

Now that he's grown
and on his own,
he lives in that zone
that's on the phone.

His Mama dear,
she's also here
to lend an ear (the one's that off the phone)
it's oh, so clear.

That this son of hers,
who was her furse,
took after her
for better or worse.

He loves, he helps, he cooks
just like Mama,
and keeps himself busy
just like he oughta'.

But busy and phone
and no one home,
is a lot like her
and the end of this Pome.

Pome August 12, 1995

But we can't stop here
without acknowledging we're
indebted to both
and glad they're a pair.

POWER

By William S. Horowitz, M.D.

The infant cries and the mother comes. In time he learns the connection and the ability to "work" his mother. Later this talent extends to "working" dolls, toys, and other adults. In this way the helpless (?) child gains a measure of magical power of his own plus capturing the power of the adult who cares. In the normal course of growing up the child gradually learns other skills, one of which is the ability to take care of himself, and the irresistible satisfaction of exercising his own real potency rises as the magical pleasure in manipulating others wanes. ("Please Mother, let me do it myself.") With this acquisition of competency comes in time a loss of interest in magic and a healthy regard for reality and limits. Not so, however, for the future career-manipulator of others, the professional politician.

Politics has been defined as the gentle art of exercising power over one's fellow man. Mindful of the potential for abuse of power, especially by the executive, our constitution provided for a system of checks and balances to prevent that abuse. Critics have noted that what this accomplishes is chiefly the paralysis of executive functioning, but to those politicians who have sought political power because of personal impotency, that fact serves as no deterrent. It is the thesis of this essay that our system of governance as evolved actually insures the acquisition and retention of power by our career politicians while it impotizes the electorate instead from performing its participating and overseeing function.

Since the actual power for self-governance resides within the mature individual in his capacity to regulate his own behavior, the citizenry has to be persuaded to relinquish this power to others, i.e., to collaborate in its own impotization. Obviously it requires persuasive motivators to induce an individual to give up his mature achievement and basic self-protectiveness, to resume a dependency on authority. This the politician accomplishes by appeals to idealism (the "American Way"), infantilism ("Take a spoonful of this, it's good for you."), and reason ("Society needs its members to collaborate in a division of labor."), to say nothing of the persuasiveness of outright intimidation or bribes.

One feels downright anti-social if he has achieved a modicum of self-governance, individual judgment, and pleasure in pursuit of free activity not harmful to others. To be a mature man simply earning his living, providing for his family, and engaging in pleasurable social and economic intercourse with his fellow man is felt to be almost anarchic, a term of undeniable opprobrium. There are thus powerful social pressures against maturation which work against self- and toward collective-governance.

But the society of competent, mature, free-standing citizens for the common weal is, or was, what the American noble experiment was all about in the Eighteenth century, an assertion of the dignity of the free citizenry in association. That was the time, of course, of the citizen-legislator, and not the professional one. What we are dealing with in the 21st century, however, should not be confused with that time, being but a faint trace of what was, a corruption of a still-inspiring ideal. Today's only relics of those days' rotating democratic responsibilities are perhaps the jury duty and the voting duty, both observed more in the breach than the practice.

Each morning newspaper carries a dose of the by-now usual political horror stories: the accumulation of campaign "war chests" by the selling of votes for money; the buying of votes of minorities by outright pandering to their special interests; the House of "Representatives" having less turnover than the Politburo; our government foregoing our founding ideals in the name of Realpolitik; and so forth. Disappointing, disillusioning, disgusting. Corruption reigns supreme and amorality wins the day. The levers of power in the society have been captured by the energetic moneyed minority to wield control over the disenfranchised majority. Representative democracy... or oligarchy?

This is what the powerful have discovered: America is a natural haven for the flourishing of the corrupt, lacking as is does the immune system, the individual defenders, to fight the power-seekers in order to regain the health of the body politic. Why? Because the citizens have been persuaded to relinquish both the legislative duty and the oversight duty to the institutions of government, which in turn have been captured and controlled by the career-manipulators.

What is to be done? Perhaps 200 years is enough of the "experiment", noble as it is, and time now for America to mature. What would this entail? Foremost would be a relinquishing of our kindergarten idealism in favor of a more mature realism, about the nature of humans and the world. An acknowledgement that this finite world and ourselves have limits would be a giant step, indeed, in our growing up.

We must acknowledge that we need to guard not only against the abuse of power of a chief executive, but anyone who is in power too long, including our local councilman. Automatic limits must be set on all governmental offices, not just the president's, to the end of enforcing the regular rotation among citizen-legislators and -executives the duties of running the government, which should remain an important but secondary function to their main lives. The acceptance of the notion of limits would also entail a realization that our economy can support only so many people, and only a small percentage of so many non-contributing people. We cannot, as a society, be all things to all people, and should not have the hubris to expect that we can or should.

This single idea, recognition of limits, to power and to our resources, can go a long way toward resuming our political maturation in the inspiring example of our forefathers, successful citizens and temporary amateur politicians all, who rebelled, remember, against another form of tyranny (unlimited power) which squelched self-government.

REFLECTIONS

CIRCA 1979.

This was to be a vignette about treating exceptional individuals. I am immediately aware of a sense of impossible difficulty, the mark of heavy resistance. Over confidential material? Perhaps, but perhaps something more. To resurrect lost relationships...how difficult for anyone, how difficult for an analyst who professionally experiences them repeatedly...how difficult for remembering such special human beings, who so enriched our lives, and frustrated us.

Here are two of the clues, already. Exceptional people pleasure us with their talents, their skills, their way of thinking and experiencing the world. They have the same to offer us personally and privately as they do professionally and publicly. When have you last been treated to a private performance of a piano concerto by a concert artist? I was, frequently, by a depressed, drugged and agoraphobic home-bound performer; concertized, that is, when he wasn't otherwise communicating with me either via his remembrances of the famous or his not inconsiderable writings. Here is what we might call the seduction of the innocent (analyst), and an important vulnerability to allow to function, I felt.

Right alongside it, however, was the resistance of the talent, its knowing effect in influencing the therapist, its protective use to prevent the development of a dependent relationship in which help could be given. I felt myself lending myself for a certain kind of first aid, to enable the artist to go on as he always had before, by himself, stimulating others.

I think with all the exceptional people with whom I have ever tried to work, no matter the field, I have come away enriched but diminished, turned away by their ultimate aloneness, stemming I am sure from a lifetime of being exceptional, being different, being alone, and learning to live in spite of it and by virtue of it. They are an exaggeration of "the children who are given to our care for only a moment".

This leads me to the great sadness in our work, with all our patients... to become deeply involved with human beings only to lose them one after another...is really a pain beyond bearing. It is not as with a professor and his students, nor a scientist with his collaborators, nor a parent with his (few) children. It happens over and over again, with dreadful regularity. An aged supervisor of mine sat with me for several years, and rarely spoke (it was rumored she did the same with her analysands). Now I understand it as an occupational disease.

What about performers, whose successful analytic and professional work culminates in their leaving, not once but regularly in the course of the therapeutic relationship? What do we do with that? After enough of it we withdraw, I think, exactly as others have done in their lives. We are no different, as desperately as we and they hope that we are.

Doctors in general, and psychoanalysts in particular, I think, are often drawn from the ranks of exceptional people also, though they don't often make their living from it, but rather in spite of it. When, on certain days of reflection, I cogitate on my chosen vocation of bare-chested head-butting against brick walls, I am aghast at the sheer unseeing dumb determination of it! (And this from someone who feels very effective...believe it or not.)

It is one thing to work with and bind the wounds of the halt and the lame and the insane and the weak and every other kind of unfortunate creature who needs us and thereby guarantees to us our importance and our value and our security and our relationships. And it is one thing to have them lined up for hours or for months in our waiting room or our waiting list. But to be an analyst to an exceptional person, or several, or many, is a fantastic adventure of excitement and despair, which can do nothing but humble one in the face of the wonders of nature.

So, my vignette today I suppose is about myself: beware the exceptional patient, for he can be a dangerous narcotic to the unsuspecting. And they don't teach that in medical school! Just clean technique so you don't get yourself infected.

Reflections

It seems then that when the exceptional patient leaves, repaired and refreshed enough to go on, perhaps we both return to our original state of aloneness, to do our creative work with the hearts and minds of men so as to bridge the gap between ourselves and all of them, to help overcome the terrible loneliness we all feel.

Perhaps we come face to face with ourselves in these encounters with these special people; not piece by piece as we explore the human condition with any patient, but with the whole gestalt of ourselves who followed another path. Here we have the psychology of the double, the terrible fascination and repulsion of seeing ourselves embodied in another, which threatens to obliterate our sense of ourselves.

The task is at bottom impossible, for them and for us, though irresistibly appealing...hence the narcotic, And, as we are used to saying, perhaps the exceptional patient only highlights and exaggerates that which can be found in the treatment of any patient...the irresistible attraction to the impossible relationship.

Is influencing another a chimera? Are we practicing a delusion? Is our work killing us? Faster than just living does?

I am not speaking in hyperbole now, but quite seriously addressing the issue of our human vulnerability, which at last we should take note of after having introduced our patients to it. The artist I speak of is dead, long before his contemporaries, and he was one of the most articulate human communicators I have been privileged to know, driven by a desperate need to reach across and over the gap between himself and the rest of the world. And my most articulate and empathic exemplar of psychoanalysis, his counterpart in almost every way, is dead, too. One is tempted to say of broken hearts. But who really knows? Perhaps we have taken on a superhuman task.

RIGHTEOUSNESS

William S. Horowitz, M.D.

9 October 2010

Uprightness, nobility, deserving and many more honorifics inure to this state of being. We should all desire this good in life.

After watching a replay of the '70s adventure of Daniel Ellsberg on TV P.O.V., and observing his gloating victory lap on stage with the complicitor New York Times, celebrating the downing of a president and ending of a war....(without, however, a mention of the millions of innocents slaughtered as a result of their action)....the formerly proud significance of the word took on an entirely different meaning when modified: self-righteousness, the smug assertion of virtue.

Whence cometh this satisfaction with one's sense of rightness? What motivates the revolutionary to take up arms against his fellow man; the flame-throwing author to write his inflammatory screed; the authoritarian to proclaim, "I know!"?

Is it the same as the scientist, pursuing a hint from his data to discover a fact of nature? Is it the theorist wondering if perhaps an idea could possibly be true? Is it your friend gently suggesting he disagrees? These seem different... human. The earlier examples reflect, however, what may be the sense of the possession of higher authority.

Whence cometh that? I'll tell you, I know, I read it in the Holy Bible, the source of the ultimate authority straight from the Lord's mouth....or so the ancient Hebrews claimed. They introduced the concept of monotheism, they patented the idea, then chose themselves to the awesome responsibility to pass judgment on the rest of humanity... so He is said to have tasked them. Revolutionaries, apostates, liberals, Jews, a motley assortment of beliefs all seem to feel missioned to identify and correct the wrongs and proclaim the right and thus lead the world.

Any reason this should prove to be irksome? Any surprise that such a posture arouses us to bristle? Any surprise holders of this attitude are universally disliked and held at a distance? What may be a surprise is that, on rare occasions, they are able to do some good for society, but I submit those rare cases take a long time to evolve...they are never revolutionary nor instantaneous, and do not respond to force, rather persuasion.

Although the Jews claim primogeniture in this department, their co-religionists that followed their lead also share the same perspective, most obvious in the case of the fundamentalists. (And in a subtle echo, the Christian churches and financial institutions seem addicted to proclaiming the title "FIRST".) As they also share the lock-step mindless loyalty of their followers, and the general opprobrium of the general public.

Is it really necessary to disclaim any slur at religion or other liberal politics? To clarify: the error is talking as though in the name of the Lord, as though he is the one.

THE SCOURGE OF THE TWENTIETH CENTURY

By William S. Horowitz, M.D.

July, 2009

Was there an epidemic that encompassed the globe and affected the world's population irretrievably? In a manner of speaking, yes, for more people and specifically men were destroyed by war and political events than ever occurred in all the preceding centuries combined. And in the absence of the men at war and need to support them, women entered the workforce in never-before-seen numbers. What were the sociological effects of this shift? Profound changes in crucial dimensions of the society ensued.

Buchanan has noted that by mid-21st century, the white race will no longer be in the majority in the Western world: they are not reproducing themselves in Europe, and just barely in America. Marriage rates are down, divorce is up, single parenthood is up, homosexuality is up...all contributing to the diminishing fecundity of the predominant society.

This phenomenon is not shared by the Moslem or Orthodox Jewish groups which are reproducing wildly wherever they live. It is characteristic of the Christian population, the majority of the Western society. But more about this later.

What happens to the children who grow up in this situation? The mothers of those children have gone to work, achieved independence from their former reliance on a husband's earnings, and in time become competitors of men in the workplace and in the home, no longer feeling the necessity of having a man in their life. The girl-children incorporate this independent attitude, and challenge the boys in all manner of activities. (Have you noticed the speed demons in traffic are often surprisingly female?) When they marry, they comfortably establish a competitive relationship with the man, not a supportive one like the one that enabled our grandparents to celebrate a 75th wedding anniversary! Rivals do not good partners make. Divorce is increasingly common, as is no more children.

What happens to the boy-children without a male model in the home? They turn to the mother for identification with the valued traits they wish to emulate, and thereby become impotized. Some marry and fail at it, some never marry, and some turn to "an alternate life-style" to satisfy their needs. And some go into government, a safe and secure sinecure for life. There they do **NOTHING** of significance, embarrassing the memory of real statesmen of the past.

Are there exceptions to this fate? Of course there are: there are many good husbands and fathers to their children, successful entrepreneurs and scientists and artists and professionals. And successful single men, too. This truth does not in any way diminish the truth of the very real demographic developments in our society...it only gauzes over the unpleasantness if one needs to deny that.

What is the connection to religion as a possible causative factor? Scholars have typified the Old Testament religions as God-centered, an all-powerful deity with punishing characteristics toward transgressors of his law. We see this especially in the Moslem religion, but Orthodox Judaism shares this same character. This may be reflected, in part, by the power collected and exercised by the Jews who are commonly accused of wanting to "take over the world". Modern bankers or money-changers may be exemplars.

What of the Christians? They have been typified by many religious scholars as having replaced the all-powerful father-deity with a forgiving son/mother paired one. (Of interest is the virginal state of the mother, supposedly un-inseminated or parthenogenetic.) Are there echoes of this arrangement in our Western society? Judge for yourself.

So, the "Eastern" societies are reproducing and developing their economies; the "Western" societies are not and in a state of rapid decline economically. What to do with this perspective? At very least, think about it. I offer no solution Perhaps all this has been fated for a very long time.

What do I call "The Scourge" ? FATHERLESS WOMEN AND MEN.

SHAME ON YOU

By William S. Horowitz, M.D.

The little child says, "The milk spilled". A bit older he says, "My fingers spilt the milk". Next, "All children do it". The still older child says, "I spilt the milk, but you made me do it". Thus the grudging acknowledgement of individual responsibility. The final goal: "I did it, I'm sorry, and I'll wipe it up".

With the current debate over de-criminalizing drug usage, we revisit the childhood grounds of evasion of culpability, with its appeal to relieve the users of blame and shift it onto others or "conditions", thus making it impossible to rectify the situation. Once the blame is permitted to be shifted, there is nothing left for the miscreants to do, while the recipients of it exert themselves ineffectually in all directions trying to "fix" that which they didn't do.

There is another social force at work here, also, in the cry for aborting the "War on Drugs". It is the same one which took hold during the Vietnam War, i.e., surrender. There are no good causes to fight for; there is no winning that is worth the cost of battle; if someone wants something bad enough, let him have it. This is the flip side of the previous ploy: no blame, no credit.

Both of these familiar childhood maneuvers grew into social movements in the second American civil war, the 1960's. The flower children attacked established societal values and institutions across the board and also, curiously enough, espoused a drug-available and pacifistic society.

The responsible majority are vulnerable to the irresponsible minority's appeal to accept blame for them, and in this indulgent society (non-indulgent ones don't have these debates) are liable to bleed themselves in the process of futile expiation. The trouble with that is, the doers of the crime, left with a sure knowledge of what they have done and its burden of shame and guilt, and also robbed of their personhood by others assuming responsibility for them, are left in a blind alley: feeling like nobody, and feeling bad. That impossible combination leads unerringly to "addiction" to the act. (One frequent reason children of prominent families go bad: they are "let off" early in their careers.)

The highest gift we as a society can give to our members is to credit all as responsible individuals who will be held accountable for their actions but also given the opportunity to "fix it". This is the "treatment" administered by any rehabilitation center which works, and those advocating "treating" the druggies should understand that this is the "medicine" dispensed at the clinics, and needed from the society.

It is at bottom a moral struggle, to help our young grow straight and mature, so that their behavior will be self-controlled and self-assured. Just imagine the incentive of individual responsibility restored, so that the one who does not work for a living, learn the language, nor observe the mores of the culture feels his own shame for himself, once again. Then we could feel our own justified pride, once again, in our society's accomplishments.

SURVIVOR GUILT

Gloria and William Horowitz
June 21, 2010

Survivor guilt, the persistent nagging feeling one should or could have done more to save the lost one. We have come to the understanding that this particular reaction is absolutely universal over the loss of a loved one, and actually may have nothing to do with the survivors actions or lack of them, or feelings about the subject. We proposed that the unconscious (read childhood past) omnipotently concludes that everything that happens is the child's doing, and so is the loved one's going away, whether by abandonment, accident, death, or suicide, it doesn't matter. That IRRATIONAL explanation is the source of survivor guilt, regardless of what may have happened in reality.

This should be public knowledge. Can there be RATIONAL regret about actual actions or lack of them? Of course, and they overlay and exaggerate the underlying feeling, but understanding the above may go a long way to absolving and forgiving the self, permitting dealing with the real. One of the most common losses in our society is divorce, loss of a mate and sometimes family, leading to endless recriminations about the other often covering feelings of guilty failure of the self.

The loss of a soldier son is likewise devastating, and there are guilty survivor reactions to that, too. Sometimes reactive defensive patriotic pride in the member's "service" can cover a persistent state of mourning, punishing and limiting the enjoyment of the survivor's remaining life. The alive one gives up his own life to join the lost one, so to speak.

The "guilties" or sense of badness seems to come from above, from a power superior to us, and indeed it is superior to the "us", emanating from the conscience or "better self" which lies in the "super"ego. WE are the source, not someone above us, and only we can forgive us, by understanding what is going on. Public knowledge could indeed help. The thinking self can disarm the reflexive self, the whole rationale for psychotherapy.

THE POLITICS OF SEX

June 5, 2010

This is an attempt to analyze (break into component parts) what occurs in the sexual act with reference to the power relationships between the partners. These are distinctly separate from but related to the biological, anatomical, humoral, and physiological aspects familiar to all.

She catches his eye. He pursues her, drawing closer. She locks him in by opening her self-containment a bit. Now excited, his urge is to get to her, to penetrate her self-control and to rupture her control over him. She responds by progressively losing her self-control and becoming excited herself. The mutually reinforce their partner's excitement, each climaxing in a total loss of self-control. After his "success," he is momentarily "spent," arousal recedes, and attraction is lost. She feels rejuvenated by confirmation of her desirability (power), regaining self-control and activity.

Power relationships between humans are rarely spoken about in scientific circles, somehow being relegated merely to a popular arena. But, in fact they are significant and possibly pre-potent in understanding both normal (as above) or pathological (as in rape/murder or child-sex predation) behavior. What has long been understood in animal societies, then phenomenon of dominance hierarchies or "pecking order," has been missing in our psychology of human behavior; freely acknowledged, however, in the realm of governance. Power = control over others = politics.

One can trace derivatives of these fundamental dynamics in the superficial social relations between the sexes (from dating to marriage), and in the family, in the workplace and in the society at large. They are tellingly clarifying to understanding both the smooth working s as well as the failures of the human social adaptation, remaining to be elaborated by students of the science.

TO BE OR NOT TO BE

William S. Horowitz, M.D.

The accession of a mixed-race, non-U.S. born son of immigrant parents to the highest office in the land has been called the first post-American President, popularly and by the cognoscenti alike, laying bare the fundamentally-flawed unconstitutional contretemps now facing this nation. This is the overwhelmingly crucial problem of our time. Less emergent but no less important is the light it sheds on the dilemma of ALL immigrant peoples to this culture, not to mention the prescience of our founding fathers.

What preoccupies the child and developing adolescent beyond all else? I submit it is the existential question of WHAT TO BE when grown. And how is it to be determined, from all the models and possibilities confronting him as he grows in his education and experience? There are multiple influences, to be sure, but perhaps unbeknownst to him and lying beneath the surface is the primordial identification with his beloved parents, often symbolized in his family name. As much as the teenager rebels and denies this heritage, it remains powerful residing in his unknown.

In the traditional and common course of events, this identification often leads to the phenomenon of "following in his father's footsteps", the ubiquitous Jones and Sons on the shop marquee. (Needless to add, we see substance-abuse and anti-social identifications as well.)

But what if the parent has not yet found a consistent identity himself to be included by his incorporating child? What if the immigrant parent was a shoemaker in the old world and comes into the new with absolutely no idea what his eventual career path may take? He may, likely will, try a variety of life-modes before settling on one at which he is successful. During this process, is he casting about for what to be, just as an adolescent newcomer to society might experience, and perhaps not unlike his own growing child who is simultaneously following his confusing path.

Not knowing what lies before him, although seeing all the possibilities, results in a kind of blindness, a psychic blindness, which fails to find a definitive focus on something or a path to that something. He is thus at the mercy of taking any random direction that presents itself, resulting in an accidental or haphazard choice. (You see everything in the jungle BUT the way to go.)

There are numerous inviting offshoots to this construction:

- How many generations does this affect: besides the first children of immigrants, what about their children, the second...and beyond?

- Does the dilemma encompass not only WHAT to be but also HOW to be? This would account for the usual social, value-system, and language inertia of newcomers here.

- What about immigrants, not from a foreign land but from the stable east coming to California? Do those children experience instability based on the unsettledness of their parents in the new environment...and does this in turn account for the rootless ness of the Western society?

- And is our president's blurred allegiances a product of doubts about his actual religion, or even moreso from both our and his not knowing WHO HE IS? (Skepticism voiced TO THIS DAY by political commentators).

Identity formation in a stable society is complex enough molded by interpersonal and intrapsychic forces and the passage of time. How much more complicated must it be in an unstable diverse globalist world ? We may be a generation of perpetual "wannabes" waiting to gel into solid citizens.

"Land of opportunity." "You can be anything you want to be ." "No old-world rigid, stratified society this." These slogans, voiced by chauvinists who see only the positives of our unorganized society, have a point to be sure. BUT, how account for those who fail to find their way altogether, or those who have finally chosen a workable path only to discover later in life an anomie and alienation stemming from a sense of inauthenticity. This may be the "opportunity" cost finally uncovered.

Immigrants typically cluster in neighborhoods where everyone is known as well as their occupation and their place in the micro-society. This supplies them with an identity that would be otherwise missing. Nowadays, in the native population we don't live in neighborhoods anymore, lacking a particular place and sense of identity amongst the larger diverse population (except for a all-encompassing national one).

There may be a special case of immigrant identity diffusion occurring in the Jewish population upon re-entry into the gentile community, from which they had been separated traditionally. Those "wandering Jews" who attempt to re-join society and assimilate may have an even harder time finding a suitable place there as a product of both internal religious strictures and external prohibitions, perpetuating their rootless status and consequent sense of alienation.

And what about the blacks, forced émigrés many generations ago, the recent influx of Mexican trespassers, and the Asians and other groups? We have taken pride in our founding heritage as a "Nation of Immigrants". Are these old- and new-comers also to be viewed as a source of strength for our society? For sure their advocates will shout a resounding YES. But can we anticipate, if it is not already readily apparent, that these peoples will have multiplied difficulties in establishing an American identity compared to those of (our) European origin. To naively ignore this is to leave our beloved country subject to unrecognizable degradation.

TO BELONG

Gloria and William Horowitz
June 27, 2010

Picture the newborn grasping his mother's finger in his fist, whilst holding her trunk with the other arm, "holding on for dear life". Shift channels and view the monkey infant clinging to his mother's fur and body as she smoothly glides through the branches. Is this the evolutionary forebear of the clinging impulse in humans (a later edition of which is seen when toddlers are first brought to school)?

If these behaviors follow emergence from the womb, when the fetus experienced total containment, they could be seen as direct resultants of the sudden birth anxiety felt at the abrupt absence of the comforting safety of being held (see La Maze). This physical insecurity is also felt as the fear of falling, that primordial state that clinging protects against.

Do these very basic human and animal behaviors, present and powerful from the very beginning of life, predictably persist during development and manifest themselves in familiar ways? Does the human want to hold on or be held? Does he seek to be one in a nexus of others, to be a member of a group, to be included, to belong? Humans, unlike tigers e.g., make groups: families, neighborhoods, cities, nations, belief creeds, country clubs, fraternities, professional and academic disciplines, and political parties, to name just a very few of the plethora of examples of human "joiningness" (Sinclair Lewis called it "Babbitry"; on Wall Street it is known as "herd mentality").

Does he likewise fear NOT being included, ranging from the independence-seeking adolescent needing popularity and acceptance now from his peer-group, to the college-age youth biting his nails over getting a bid from a fraternity, to a grown man pleading to be hired by the prestigious firm? And may he feel not fully accepted in his own family by accidents of birth date, sibling order, parenting problems, dissolution by divorce, and a multitude of possible other factors?

Is it conceivable that he is continuously concerned about being properly included, feeling left out and seeking the remedy of joining yet another group? Does the newly-emergent fledgling from the family naturally gravitate toward establishing one of his own? Do humans in general graduate from group to group to sustain the feeling of being held? Is the loner who doesn't follow this pattern, is he one who was never held in the first place?

Perhaps the near-universal complaint of feeling unwanted, justified by a panoply of situations, real or imagined that may be only rationalizations, arises from an underlying basic primordial fear in all of us...as we vainly attempt to identify the reasons and detoxify them with "therapy". Could it be this FEAR of being OUT that impels us to be ever more IN?

But groups are but a derivative or substitute for two individuals, the originals in the equation. Being accepted by one is being loved; wanting to hold is the impulse toward the beloved. Seeking love is searching to be in the arms of someone. The loss of one formerly loving and beloved is experienced as devastating grief, the return to the painful aloneness of not being held. Love IS, then, the original belonging...which we never cease trying to recapture.

WOMEN

William S. Horowitz, M.D.
May 27Th 2010

The first human the infant sees is his mother, the adult who gave rise to him, nurtured him, and protectively raised him to adulthood. This disparity between consummate power and utter helplessness is the indelible template governing all subsequent relations between the sexes, bar none. THE WOMAN HAS THE POWER and she knows it, as revealed in the adage "He pursues her until she captures him". The man, in reaction to this, vainly tries to assert his over hers. The female infant, of course, becomes the woman in time.

Our society is replete with examples, if "proof" you require. Let us start with the beginning: who gets down on his knees to beg her favors? Before that, who seduces whom? Who seeks another partner when his is busy birthing and raising? Who lives longer? Who risks all, including his life, for the love of whom?

To those "feminists" who demur, how come the male-wannabes seek empowerment from their "unequal" weakened position? Perhaps the mysteriously-motivated crime of rape, previously ascribed to either sexual or aggressive impulses, can finally be empathically understood as an attempt to over-power the stronger by the weaker. Perhaps the time-honored suppression of the Islamic female (replete with a mathematical weighting of four of the one equaling one of the other) is another unrecognized testament to the thesis – typically disguised as it's opposite.

We are familiar with the biological irrelevance of the male in reproduction by the phenomenon of parthenogenesis, whereby the egg membrane being penetrated by any mechanical means will initiate cell division, the sperm contents only providing another DNA supply that contributes variation but is not strictly necessary. The Catholic myth of VIRGIN BIRTH is an interesting lay recognition of this possibility, but is only a myth; Jesus received his y-chromosome from his father, not his mother.

Society's' attempts to trumpet the "fact" of male superiority is another such myth: its manifestations are too numerous and familiar to enumerate here. It is the apparent puzzling observations noted above which give the lie to it. One may wonder, rather, why the denial of the obvious? Is the realization of the difference in the genders' biological significance intolerable; his optional family role; his borderline dispensability?

Actually, he makes the signal contribution of raising the biological kingdom from an asexual to a sexual level, providing the reproductive process a robustness not found in the animal realm of clones. Thus, his value and significance is found in his jeans (g..), not his power. What is in his power is only to contribute, or not contribute, to the species, a choice made too often these days by an increasing cohort of males. It is a demographic fact that the population reproduction rate is falling below maintenance all over the Western world, whilst male homosexuality is either increasing in incidence or becoming more apparent. This societal development may thus be, not as suspected a product of unknown toxic contamination in the environment, but rather as the eventual emergence of the underlying biological reality.

A cynic might observe that the men are turning into women, possibly enhancing this view.

www.ingramcontent.com/pod-product-compliance
Lightning Source LLC
Chambersburg PA
CBHW030002190526
45157CB00014B/84